NATIONAL ACADEMIES *Sciences Engineering Medicine*

NATIONAL ACADEMIES PRESS
Washington, DC

Vaccine Risk Monitoring and Evaluation at the Centers for Disease Control and Prevention

Jane E. Henney, Kathleen Stratton, Ogan K. Kumova, and Dara Ancona
Editors

Committee to Review the Centers for Disease Control and Prevention's COVID-19 Vaccine Safety Research and Communications

Board on Population Health and Public Health Practice

Health and Medicine Division

Consensus Study Report

NATIONAL ACADEMIES PRESS 500 Fifth Street, NW Washington, DC 20001

This activity was supported by a contract between the National Academy of Sciences and the Centers for Disease Control and Prevention (#75D30121D11240-75D30123F0002). Any opinions, findings, conclusions, or recommendations expressed in this publication do not necessarily reflect the views of any organization or agency that provided support for the project.

International Standard Book Number-13: 978-0-309-53979-1
Digital Object Identifier: https://doi.org/10.17226/29240

This publication is available from the National Academies Press, 500 Fifth Street, NW, Keck 360, Washington, DC 20001; (800) 624-6242; http://www.nap.nationalacademies.org.

The manufacturer's authorized representative in the European Union for product safety is Authorised Rep Compliance Ltd., Ground Floor, 71 Lower Baggot Street, Dublin D02 P593 Ireland; www.arccompliance.com.

Copyright 2025 by the National Academy of Sciences. National Academies of Sciences, Engineering, and Medicine and National Academies Press and the graphical logos for each are all trademarks of the National Academy of Sciences. All rights reserved.

Printed in the United States of America.

Suggested citation: National Academies of Sciences, Engineering, and Medicine. 2025. *Vaccine risk monitoring and evaluation at the Centers for Disease Control and Prevention.* Washington, DC: National Academies Press. https://doi.org/10.17226/29240.

The **National Academy of Sciences** was established in 1863 by an Act of Congress, signed by President Lincoln, as a private, nongovernmental institution to advise the nation on issues related to science and technology. Members are elected by their peers for outstanding contributions to research. Dr. Marcia McNutt is president.

The **National Academy of Engineering** was established in 1964 under the charter of the National Academy of Sciences to bring the practices of engineering to advising the nation. Members are elected by their peers for extraordinary contributions to engineering. Dr. Tsu-Jae Liu is president.

The **National Academy of Medicine** (formerly the Institute of Medicine) was established in 1970 under the charter of the National Academy of Sciences to advise the nation on medical and health issues. Members are elected by their peers for distinguished contributions to medicine and health. Dr. Victor J. Dzau is president.

The three Academies work together as the **National Academies of Sciences, Engineering, and Medicine** to provide independent, objective analysis and advice to the nation and conduct other activities to solve complex problems and inform public policy decisions. The National Academies also encourage education and research, recognize outstanding contributions to knowledge, and increase public understanding in matters of science, engineering, and medicine.

Learn more about the National Academies of Sciences, Engineering, and Medicine at **www.nationalacademies.org**.

Consensus Study Reports published by the National Academies of Sciences, Engineering, and Medicine document the evidence-based consensus on the study's statement of task by an authoring committee of experts. Reports typically include findings, conclusions, and recommendations based on information gathered by the committee and the committee's deliberations. Each report has been subjected to a rigorous and independent peer-review process and it represents the position of the National Academies on the statement of task.

Proceedings published by the National Academies of Sciences, Engineering, and Medicine chronicle the presentations and discussions at a workshop, symposium, or other event convened by the National Academies. The statements and opinions contained in proceedings are those of the participants and are not endorsed by other participants, the planning committee, or the National Academies.

Rapid Expert Consultations published by the National Academies of Sciences, Engineering, and Medicine are authored by subject-matter experts on narrowly focused topics that can be supported by a body of evidence. The discussions contained in rapid expert consultations are considered those of the authors and do not contain policy recommendations. Rapid expert consultations are reviewed by the institution before release.

For information about other products and activities of the National Academies, please visit www.nationalacademies.org/about/whatwedo.

COMMITTEE TO REVIEW THE CENTERS FOR DISEASE CONTROL AND PREVENTION'S COVID-19 VACCINE SAFETY RESEARCH AND COMMUNICATIONS

JANE E. HENNEY (*Chair*)
DENISE H. CHRYSLER, Network for Public Health Law
LAWRENCE DEYTON, George Washington University
FRANCISCO GARCÍA, University of Arizona
KRISHIKA A. GRAHAM, New York City Department of Health and Mental Hygiene
MARIE R. GRIFFIN, Vanderbilt University Medical Center
PERRY N. HALKITIS, Rutgers University
SONIA HERNÁNDEZ-DÍAZ, Harvard T.H. Chan School of Public Health
ALI S. KHAN, University of Nebraska Medical Center
DANIELLA MEEKER, Yale University
GLEN NOWAK, University of Georgia
OLAYINKA SHIYANBOLA, University of Michigan College of Pharmacy
LILLIE D. WILLIAMSON, University of Wisconsin–Madison

National Academy of Medicine Fellow

JENNIFER BACCI, University of Washington School of Pharmacy

Study Staff

KATHLEEN STRATTON, Study Director, Scholar
OGAN K. KUMOVA, Program Officer
DARA ANCONA, Associate Program Officer
KATIE PETERSON, Senior Program Assistant (*from December 2024*)
OLIVIA LOIBNER, Senior Program Assistant (*until August 2024*)
ROSE MARIE MARTINEZ, Senior Board Director, Board on Population Health and Public Health Practice

Reviewers

This Consensus Study Report was reviewed in draft form by individuals chosen for their diverse perspectives and technical expertise. The purpose of this independent review is to provide candid and critical comments that will assist the National Academies of Sciences, Engineering, and Medicine in making each published report as sound as possible and to ensure that it meets the institutional standards for quality, objectivity, evidence, and responsiveness to the study charge. The review comments and draft manuscript remain confidential to protect the integrity of the deliberative process.

We thank the following individuals for their review of this report:

JOAN DUWVE, San Joaquin County Health Department
KATHRYN M. EDWARDS, Vanderbilt University
CLAIRE HANNAN, Association of Immunization Managers
GRACE M. LEE, Stanford University
WALTER ORENSTEIN, Emory University
RICHARD PLATT, Harvard Medical School
SASKIA R. POPESCU, University of Maryland
ARTHUR L. REINGOLD, University of California, Berkeley
DANIEL SALMON, Johns Hopkins University
STEPHANIE SILVERA, Montclair State University

Although the reviewers listed above provided many constructive comments and suggestions, they were not asked to endorse the conclusions or recommendations of this report nor did they see the final draft before its release. The review of this report was overseen by **CATHERINE E. WOTECKI,** Iowa State University, and **PAUL A. VOLBERDING,** University of California, San Francisco. They responsible for making certain that an independent examination of this report was carried out in accordance with the standards of the National Academies and that all review comments were carefully considered. Responsibility for the final content rests entirely with the authoring committee and the National Academies.

Acknowledgments

The Committee to Review the Centers for Disease Control and Prevention's COVID-19 Vaccine Safety Research and Communications and the Board on Population Health and Public Health Practice staff would like to thank the many individuals who contributed to the development of this report.

The committee acknowledges the support of staff in the Health and Medicine Division of the National Academies of Sciences, Engineering, and Medicine, particularly the guidance and efforts of Kathleen Stratton (study director), Ogan Kumova (program officer), and Dara Ancona (associate program officer), whose work in gathering research, organizing meetings, and shaping, editing, and fact-checking this report was invaluable. The committee also extends its appreciation to Katie Peterson for her support with meeting logistics and manuscript preparation. Rose Marie Martinez (Senior Board Director, Board on Population Health and Public Health Practice) provided essential guidance to both the committee and staff throughout the process.

The committee would also like to thank Dr. John Su, Ms. Julianne Gee, and Dr. Daniel Jernigan for their informative presentations about the committee's charge and the current structure and role of the Immunization Safety Office and its safety monitoring systems. Additionally, the committee thanks invited speakers Dr. Reed Tuckson, Dr. Malia Jones, and Dr. Scott Razan for sharing their perspectives on the challenges and opportunities for research and communication related to vaccine safety.

Additional support for this report was provided by Misrak Dabi and Greysi Patton (Finance Business Partners), Crysti Park (Program Coordinator), Lori Brenig (Editorial Projects Coordinator), Taryn Young (Report Review Associate), Leslie Sim (Senior Report Review Officer), Marguerite Romatelli (Communications Specialist), Amber McLaughlin (Director of Communications), and Tasha Bigelow (copyeditor), all of whom offered outstanding assistance during each phase of the study.

Finally, the committee expresses its gratitude to the members of the public who shared their insights via email correspondence and public comments, and to those who participated in the key informant interviews, which informed the committee's work and enriched the report.

Contents

ACRONYMS AND ABBREVIATIONS — xv

SUMMARY — 1

1 INTRODUCTION — 15
Vaccine Safety Assessment, 16
CDC ISO, 17
Committee Approach to the Statement of Task, 20
Report Structure and Terminology, 27
References, 28

2 DATA MONITORING AND EVALUATION — 29
ISO Monitoring and Evaluation/Assessment Systems, 31
Major Methodologic Strengths/Limitations of Findings/
    Safety Assessments from Each of the Major Systems, 39
Timeliness and Completeness of Signals, 47
Opportunity/Attention Costs, 52
Additional Unpublished, Real-Time Findings/Safety
    Assessments, 56
Conclusion, 57
References, 60

3 COMMUNICATIONS 71
Public Health Communications, 71
Vaccine and Vaccination-Related Benefit–Risk
  Communication, 73
Vaccine Safety Communications at the Centers for Disease
  Control and Prevention (CDC), 75
Communications During the PHE, 77
Assessment of CDC Vaccine Risk Communications, 84
Conclusion, 91
References, 93

4 CONCLUSIONS AND RECOMMENDATIONS 97
Conclusions, 98
Recommendations, 99
Public Health Emergencies, 107
Concluding Thoughts, 108
References, 108

APPENDIXES
A	Committee Member and Staff Biographies	111
B	Public Meeting Agendas	121
C	Westat Key Informant Interviews Findings Report	125
D	Case Studies	181
E	Catalog of Data-Driven Literature from CDC Vaccine Safety Monitoring	209

Boxes, Figures, and Tables

BOXES

1-1 Statement of Task, 16
1-2 Emergency Use Authorization (EUA), 18
1-3 Key Functions of the Immunization Safety Office (ISO), 21
1-4 Salient Points from Public Comment, 24

3-1 CDC Vaccine Safety Communication Efforts, 77

4-1 Principles of a Robust Vaccine Risk Monitoring and Evaluation System That Merits the Nation's Trust, 100

FIGURES

S-1 Committee's understanding of ISO workflow, 4

1-1 Committee's understanding of ISO workflow, 22

3-1 CDC vaccine safety key audiences and communications, 78
3-2 CDC vaccine safety communication activities timeline during the public health emergency, 79
3-3 CDC vaccine safety communications routine clearance process vs. clearance process during the COVID public health emergency, 83

TABLES

S-1   ISO-Affiliated COVID Vaccine Risk Monitoring Systems, 5

1-1   Vaccine Offices in the Department of Health and Human Services, 23

2-1   Key Strengths and Limitations of CDC COVID Vaccine Safety Surveillance Systems, 40
2-2   Description of Non-CDC COVID Vaccine Safety Data Sources Relevant to ISO, 43
2-3   Cross-System Summary of Major COVID Vaccine Safety Signals, Principal Findings, and Surveillance Periods, 48
2-4   Selected COVID Vaccine-Safety Signals—Timeline from Initial VaST Review to Public Disclosure, Peer-Reviewed Evidence, and Action, 58

3-1   Publicly Available CDC Vaccine Safety Communications, 80
3-2   CDC COVID-19 Vaccine Safety Task Force Teams, 82

Acronyms and Abbreviations

AAP	American Academy of Pediatrics
ACCV	Advisory Committee on Childhood Vaccines
ACIP	Advisory Committee on Immunization Practice
AE	adverse event
AEFI	adverse event following immunization
AESI	adverse event of special interest
BEST	Biologics Effectiveness and Safety
CBER	Center for Biologics Evaluation and Research
CBO	community-based organization
CDC	Centers for Disease Control and Prevention
CISA	Clinical Immunization Safety Assessment
CMS	Centers for Medicare & Medicaid Services
COCA	Clinician Outreach and Communication Activity
CVST	cerebral venous sinus thrombosis
DHQP	Division of Healthcare Quality and Promotion
DoD	Department of Defense
DUA	data-use agreement
EHR	electronic health record
EPI-X	Epidemic Information Exchange
EUA	Emergency Use Authorization

FDA	Food and Drug Administration
FTE	full-time employee
GACVS	Global Advisory Committee on Vaccine Safety
GBS	Guillan-Barré Syndrome
GVDN	Global Vaccine Data Network
HCP	health care provider
HHS	Department of Health and Human Services
HRSA	Health Resources and Services Administration
IHS	Indian Health Service
IIS	Immunization Information System
IRB	Institutional Review Board
ISO	Immunization Safety Office
MMWR	*Morbidity and Mortality Weekly Report*
NCEZID	National Center for Emerging and Zoonotic Infectious Diseases
NCIRD	National Center for Immunization and Respiratory Diseases
NCVIA	National Childhood Vaccine Injury Act
NIH	National Institutes of Health
NIP	National Immunization Program
NVAC	National Vaccine Advisory Committee
NVSS	National Vital Statistics System
OWS	Operation Warp Speed
PHE	public health emergency
PREP	Public Readiness and Emergency Preparedness
PRR	proportional reporting ratio
RCA	rapid-cycle analysis
SPHA	state and territorial health agency
TTS	thrombosis with thrombocytopenia syndrome
VA	Department of Veterans Affairs
VAERS	Vaccine Adverse Event Reporting System
VaST	Vaccine Safety Technical Work Group

VICP	Vaccine Injury Compensation Program
VIS	Vaccine Information Statement
VRBPAC	Vaccines and Related Biological Products Advisory Committee
VSD	Vaccine Safety Datalink
VST	Vaccine Safety Team
VTF	Vaccine Task Force

Summary[1]

The Centers for Disease Control and Prevention's (CDC's) Immunization Safety Office (ISO) is responsible for studying vaccine risks once vaccines are administered to the public. ISO was already a federal focal point for vaccine risk evaluation when the COVID pandemic emerged and the Secretary of Health and Human Services (HHS) declared a nationwide public health emergency (PHE). By the end of 2020, vaccines were available to the general public due to Operation Warp Speed and a Food and Drug Administration (FDA) regulatory pathway called Emergency Use Authorization.

ISO is within the Division of Healthcare Quality Promotion of the National Center for Emerging and Zoonotic Infectious Diseases and administratively and organizationally separate from offices in the National Center for Immunization and Respiratory Diseases that support vaccine use. During the PHE, ISO underwent temporary restructuring as part of CDC's comprehensive response. Its vaccine specialists were integrated into the broader COVID-19 Vaccine Task Force, enabling rapid scale-up of monitoring and evaluation capabilities by leveraging both established systems and novel platforms for timely assessments of vaccine risks.

Vaccines have long been essential in public health, recognized as one of the most significant achievements of the 20th century. Unlike treatments to manage infectious diseases, vaccines prepare the immune system to prevent or mitigate infections and are often administered well before potential disease exposure. Given their preventive nature, their importance is often

---

[1] References are not included in this summary; citations are in the report chapters.

overlooked and may create unique ethical considerations, especially since vaccination decisions are sometimes mandated in certain settings, such as schools or health facilities. Despite rigorous scientific scrutiny through clinical trials and ongoing postmarket safety monitoring, the COVID vaccine became suspect to some because of public confusion, concern, and mistrust about recommended public health measures employed during the PHE, including vaccines.

STATEMENT OF TASK

CDC commissioned the National Academies of Sciences, Engineering, and Medicine to undertake a comprehensive evaluation of ISO. An ad hoc committee was tasked with conducting a thorough assessment of ISO's statistical and epidemiological methods in vaccine risk monitoring and evaluation, including detailed scrutiny of processes designed to detect, evaluate, and report potential problems associated with COVID vaccines, which encompassed systems like the Vaccine Adverse Event Reporting System (VAERS) and Vaccine Safety Datalink (VSD).

Critically, the committee was also charged with evaluating CDC's external communication strategies targeted toward diverse audiences, including health professionals, public health authorities, and the general public. The evaluation involved reviewing communication practices and analyzing content.

Additionally, the committee's mandate included providing actionable recommendations designed to sustain and enhance ISO's vaccine risk monitoring and communication systems. These recommendations aim to ensure the robustness, scientific rigor, transparency, and responsiveness of ISO's activities, positioning it to more effectively manage future vaccine risk[2] monitoring and public communication during ongoing and emergent public health initiatives.

COMMITTEE APPROACH

The committee conducted its review of ISO's vaccine risk monitoring, evaluation, and communication practices using diverse and complementary approaches. This included a detailed analysis of ISO's systems and publications for effectiveness in identifying, assessing, and communicating about vaccine risks.

The committee held multiple public meetings to gather information from ISO, health professionals, and researchers that explored ISO functioning

---

[2] The committee uses the word "risk" to indicate serious, untoward health consequences and avoids the word "safety" because many infer from it a complete lack of risks or a balance of risks and benefits.

and strategies to study and communicate with historically marginalized populations that might be skeptical of vaccination. A targeted public comment sessions addressed criteria for studies of vaccine risks, strategies for improving research, communication practices, and methods to bolster public confidence.

The committee also commissioned confidential key informant interviews with experts in vaccine safety, epidemiology, public health communication, and policy. These yielded qualitative insights and actionable recommendations. In addition, the committee developed case studies analyzing ISO's handling of specific vaccine risk issues, which informed its final recommendations by illustrating both strengths and gaps in current practices.

Building on this extensive methodological review, public engagement, expert consultation, and case analysis, the committee turned its focus to evaluating the specific systems and practices ISO employed during the COVID pandemic. It did so by examining ISO public scientific reporting, such as presentations at federal advisory committee meetings and scientific publications, and CDC webpages. The following findings highlight how ISO's key monitoring and evaluation platforms functioned in practice, the strengths and limitations of its risk assessments, and the communication challenges that emerged in a rapidly evolving public health landscape. Figure S-1 shows the committee's understanding of ISO's workflow.

Monitoring and Evaluation Systems

ISO leveraged a suite of systems to monitor vaccine risks, including VAERS, VSD, Clinical Immunization Safety Assessment network (CISA), V-safe, and the COVID-19 Vaccine Pregnancy Registry. These platforms formed a deliberately overlapping architecture—early signal detection, rapid active analysis, clinical assessments, near-real-time self-reporting, and longitudinal follow-up for sensitive populations—so that no single evidence stream bore the entire burden of risk assessment and layered and comprehensive monitoring was possible. Table S-1 presents a quick snapshot of the five CDC-affiliated systems that formed the backbone of COVID vaccine safety monitoring.

VAERS, a joint CDC-FDA passive reporting system, provided early signals, though it was limited by underreporting and lack of control groups. For example, it produced the first U.S. alerts of myocarditis after mRNA vaccination in May 2021, prompting deeper analysis in VSD.

VSD offered rapid assessments and in-depth targeted analysis using electronic health records. Weekly rapid-cycle analyses (RCAs) across roughly 12 million patients quantified the myocarditis incidence at about

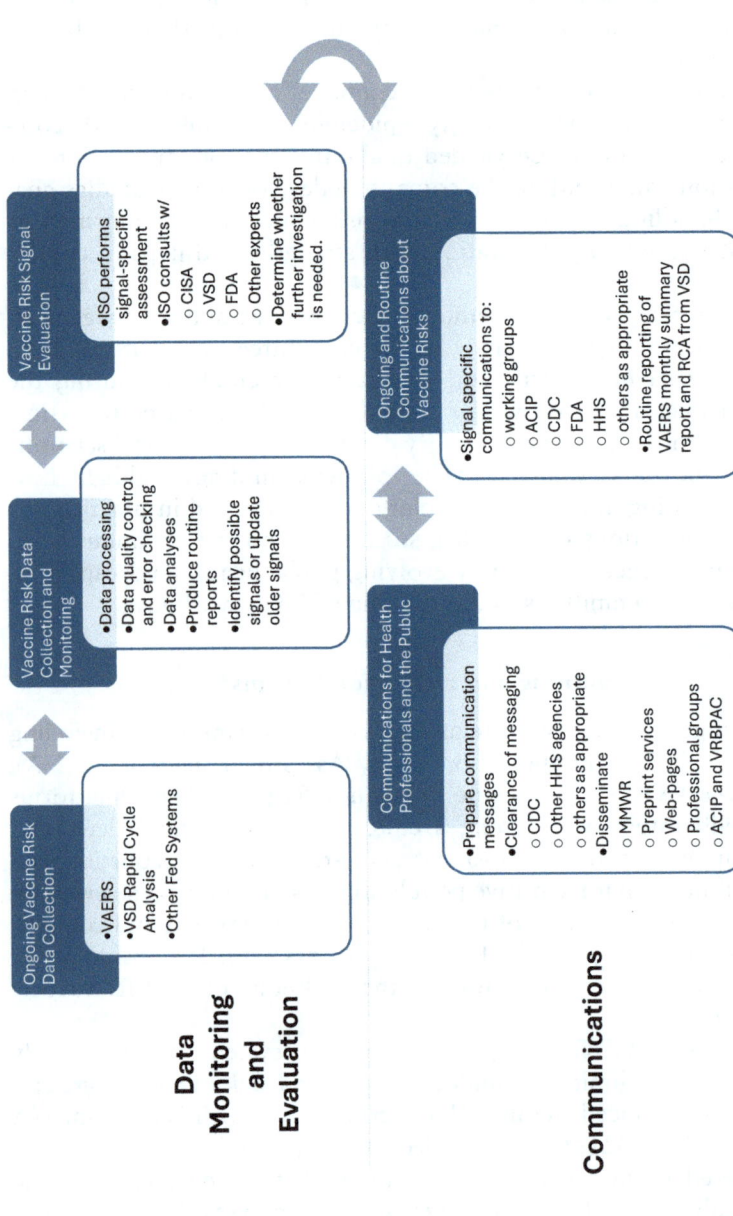

FIGURE S-1 Committee's understanding of ISO workflow.
NOTES: Passive and active data streams (e.g., Vaccine Adverse Event Reporting System, Vaccine Safety Datalink) move through sequential processing and signal-evaluation steps, then feed into cleared messages and routine updates for clinicians, partners, and the public. Bidirectional arrows highlight continuous feedback between monitoring and communication functions.

TABLE S-1 ISO-Affiliated COVID Vaccine Risk Monitoring Systems

System	Managed by	Description and Data Source
VAERS	ISO & FDA (joint)	Passive, nationwide early-warning signal detection through clinician, patient, and manufacturer reports
VSD	ISO + 13 integrated health care organizations	Active surveillance using electronic health record data for RCAs and multisite cohort studies
V-safe	ISO	Smartphone-based, voluntary postvaccination check-ins providing near-real-time reactogenicity trends
COVID-19 Vaccine Pregnancy Registry	ISO	Subregistry of pregnant V-safe participants with medical-record follow-up to track maternal and infant outcomes
CISA	ISO-coordinated network of seven academic medical centers	Expert clinical consultation and mechanistic research on rare or complex adverse events

NOTE: CISA = Clinical Immunization Safety Assessment; FDA = Food and Drug Administration; ISO = Immunization Safety Office; RSA = rapid-cycle analysis; VAERS = Vaccine Adverse Event Reporting System; VSD = Vaccine Safety Datalink.

6.5 cases per million second doses among 12–39-year-olds within 6 weeks of the initial VAERS signal.

CISA contributed expert consultations and in-depth evaluations of individual reporting serious and unusual reactions, though its case-specific approach limits generalizability. Expanded virtual case conferences in 2021 helped elucidate the pathophysiology of thrombosis with thrombocytopenia syndrome (TTS) linked to the Janssen vaccine, informing the Advisory Committee on Immunization Practices (ACIP) decision to recommend the April 2021 temporary pause in use of that vaccine.

The newly launched V-safe system captured real-time self-reported data on postvaccination effects, identifying trends like menstrual irregularities. With 9.3 million enrollees, it flagged those menstrual cycle changes in late 2021 and triggered a dedicated cohort study in VSD, but its self-reported nature and lack of clinical validation remain limitations.

The COVID-19 Vaccine Pregnancy Registry addressed a critical data gap. An interim analysis published in April 2021 showed a 12 percent spontaneous-abortion rate—comparable to background—shaping obstetric recommendations and easing early concerns.

In addition to CDC's systems, a network of external vaccine safety surveillance platforms operated by agencies like FDA, the Centers for Medicare & Medicaid Services (CMS), the Department of Veterans Affairs, the Indian Health Service, and vaccine manufacturers contributed complementary datasets, methods, and populations to COVID vaccine safety monitoring. These systems helped triangulate evidence, extended surveillance beyond CDC-covered populations, and enabled early signal identification across diverse geographies and contexts.

Timeliness and completeness of signal evaluation were further strengthened by the Vaccine Safety Technical (VaST) Work Group, which met weekly during the first 18 months of the vaccine rollout and monthly thereafter. Its rapid review—often within days of the first doses administered—enabled ACIP and CDC to issue interim clinical guidance on anaphylaxis, myocarditis, TTS, pregnancy safety, and other adverse events of special interest. This prespecified outcome list gave the program an analytically focused backbone, but it remained flexible: unexpected conditions, such as menstrual changes or tinnitus, were added as public concern arose. Where data were sparse, VaST and ISO triaged resources—a quick descriptive VAERS analysis for early context while labor-intensive VSD chart reviews ran in parallel. These efforts were facilitated by temporary data-use agreements that expanded access to vaccination data and enabled timely linkage to health outcomes. However, without a permanent national reporting infrastructure, fragmentation across state systems and inconsistent standards continued to hinder comprehensive, long-term surveillance.

Timeliness brings unavoidable opportunity costs. Every new investigation diverted epidemiologists, statisticians, and clinician reviewers from other monitoring tasks, yet the criteria for elevating, deferring, or ceasing work on a specific signal were not fully explained publicly. Greater transparency around those prioritization decisions and the resource implication across safety systems would bolster confidence in ISO's capacity to target effort where it yields greater public health return.

Despite the robustness and thoroughness of ISO's activities, challenges remained, particularly regarding clear communication of findings to health professionals and the public. Translating RCA statistical output into plain language and actionable guidance proved difficult: weekly myocarditis risk estimates, for example, were posted in ACIP slide decks long before they appeared in peer-reviewed journals, leaving frontline clinicians to interpret evolving numbers without clear context or caveats. Communication issues occasionally undermined the extensive scientific efforts undertaken to assess vaccine risks comprehensively. Additionally, ISO's scientific publications and communications from CDC consistently included strong messages about vaccine benefits, fueling perceptions of bias.

The COVID pandemic underscored ISO's critical role in vaccine risk monitoring and evaluation, demonstrating the importance of integrating multiple complementary monitoring systems to rapidly and accurately assess vaccine risks. This integrated approach not only facilitated immediate public health responses but also established a strong foundation for future vaccine risk monitoring. Sustaining this level of performance will require durable governance structures and improved coordination across federal agencies. While ISO partnered effectively with organizations like the National Institutes of Health, CMS, and FDA, the lack of centralized coordination with other state and local agencies limited alignment of analytic priorities and data integration. Enhancing transparency, clearly distinguishing ISO's role from efforts to encourage vaccination, and continuously refining methodologies will be essential to maintain public trust and effectively address emerging vaccine risk challenges.

Communication Challenges and Public Trust

CDC has been a pivotal institution in addressing public health crises, with vaccine effectiveness and risk communication becoming particularly crucial during the unprecedented PHE; it developed and implemented comprehensive strategies to communicate clearly and effectively about the benefits and risks associated with the vaccines. However, the complexity and evolving nature of the pandemic introduced significant challenges, affecting how health professionals, policy makers, and the general public received and acted upon information.

At the onset of the pandemic, CDC recognized the necessity for transparent and timely communication. Despite extensive communication efforts, vaccine hesitancy persisted due to concerns about the novelty of the mRNA technology, FDA's regulatory approach, uncertainties about potential side effects, trust in authorities, and skepticism about effectiveness.

CDC's communication strategies were multifaceted, designed to meet the distinct informational needs of various stakeholders, such as health professionals, policy makers, public health officials, and the broader community. CDC employed a variety of tools, including ACIP meetings, Clinician Outreach and Communication Activity calls, *Morbidity and Mortality Weekly Reports* (MMWRs), and extensive online content. These platforms provided continuous updates and detailed discussions of vaccine risk data, monitoring results, and emerging scientific findings. For instance, ACIP meetings, usually three times a year, increased dramatically to 27 public sessions during the PHE, underscoring the urgency and importance of the vaccine risk discourse.

Despite these robust mechanisms, areas of communication fell short of fully engaging and adequately informing all intended audiences. One primary concern was the overly technical language in many CDC communications. The agency often presumed a baseline understanding of scientific terminology and vaccine risk principles. This posed challenges for not only the general public but also many health professionals, who, despite their backgrounds, may not have specialized expertise in vaccine risk communication. It limited the accessibility and effectiveness of some of CDC's critical risk messages. State and local health departments were often better positioned than federal agencies to engage trusted community messengers and respond in real time. Strengthening the complementary roles of CDC and these local entities—and tailoring communications to local needs—can enhance message effectiveness and credibility.

Another significant issue was the inconsistent use of and lack of clear definitions for important terms, like "risk," "adverse events," "adverse events of special interest," "side effects," and "safety signals." Without clear, uniform definitions, these terms became sources of potential misunderstanding and confusion, particularly when comparing different vaccine risks. For example, risk estimates were sometimes presented in vague terms, like "higher" or "most frequently," without precise quantification or context, which could lead to misinterpreting actual risks.

The communications occasionally included broad, generalized statements, such as references to "the most intense safety monitoring in U.S. history," without adequate supporting details about what precisely made it more rigorous. Such broad statements, without substantive backing, risked undermining public trust by appearing overly promotional rather than factual. Further complicating the situation, structural issues with CDC's web presence impacted how easily individuals could locate relevant information. The content often lacked clear organization, making it challenging to discern whether it was intended for health professionals, public health officials, or the general public. This structural confusion was compounded by multiple pages with overlapping or redundant content, hindering effective navigation and engagement.

In addressing these shortcomings, CDC could significantly enhance its communications by adopting clearer, more accessible language and structured, consistent terminology. This approach would not oversimplify the information but instead ensure that scientific findings were effectively translated into actionable and understandable messages for all audiences. Detailed explanations of the methods and rationale behind risk monitoring efforts would reinforce credibility and facilitate greater public trust.

Further challenges to effective communication arose from procedural and structural constraints. During the pandemic, the federal clearance process—designed to ensure message consistency—sometimes delayed or constrained the dissemination of risk findings, particularly when research involved external collaborators. These delays, combined with the predominantly unidirectional nature of vaccine safety communications, limited opportunities for timely public engagement and contributed to perceptions of opacity. Integrating more accessible formats—such as interactive explainers, visual dashboards, and moderated forums—alongside traditional outlets, like the MMWR, would improve transparency and support bidirectional communication with both professional and public audiences.

CONCLUSIONS AND RECOMMENDATIONS

During the PHE, ISO staff demonstrated commendable agility by quickly adapting existing systems and developing new tools, such as V-safe. The rapid deployment and management of risk monitoring systems facilitated an unprecedented volume of high-quality, timely data on vaccine risks. The meticulous and transparent presentation of these findings, including at open federal advisory committee meetings, was instrumental in guiding immediate public health responses. However, ISO's ability to respond was also constrained by structural limitations in the U.S. surveillance ecosystem, many of which fell outside its direct purview. Fragmented data systems, lack of real-time data exchange, and inconsistent technical standards impeded comprehensive analysis. Additionally, the absence of transparent criteria for prioritizing safety signals meant that emerging public concerns—such as menstrual changes—often outpaced analytic response. Addressing these gaps will require a clear framework for signal prioritization and investment in interoperable infrastructure that can support timely, cross-system risk detection.

However, despite ISO's robust scientific processes, the office faces ongoing challenges, particularly concerning public trust and understanding. These challenges often arise from the perceived overlap between vaccine risk monitoring activities and broader vaccination efforts at CDC, which some critics argue undermines ISO's perceived impartiality. This perception can lead to skepticism among segments of the public, complicating efforts to communicate scientifically grounded vaccine risk assessments effectively.

Conclusions

Based on its comprehensive evaluation—including analysis of monitoring and evaluation systems, stakeholder input, expert interviews, and communication products and practices—the committee concluded that ISO carried out scientifically robust, timely, and effective vaccine risk monitoring throughout the COVID pandemic. Its proactive identification and response to emerging vaccine risk concerns informed critical public health decisions. The following conclusions summarize key strengths.

Conclusion 4-1: ISO has played an important role performing and communicating about rigorous vaccine risk monitoring and evaluation.

Conclusion 4-2: In response to the COVID public health emergency declaration, ISO staff and systems produced and communicated an impressive quantity of timely, important, and high-quality monitoring, evaluation, and communication about COVID vaccine risks.

Despite these accomplishments, the committee identified ongoing challenges related to public trust, transparency, and the perception of ISO's independence. The perceived overlap between ISO's risk monitoring activities and CDC's broader efforts to encourage vaccine use continues to raise concerns about the impartiality and objectivity of risk assessments, negatively affecting public confidence in and use of vaccines.

Conclusion 4-3: Trust in ISO as a credible source of vaccine risk information is affected by the intersection and interaction with CDC and other governmental efforts to foster vaccination. ISO currently lacks the organizational independence and resources to directly disseminate its information to health professionals, policy makers, and the public.

Recommendations

The committee does not want its focus on the risks of COVID vaccines to detract from the overwhelming evidence of their benefits. One way to increase use of vaccines, and therefore the benefits, is to increase understanding of and confidence in federal studies of vaccine risks. Recognizing the significance of ISO's role, the committee proposed critical recommendations aimed at enhancing its capabilities and supporting its capacity.[3] These focus on five core principles crucial for a robust vaccine risk monitoring system that merits the nation's trust: relevance, credibility, data stewardship, continuous improvement, and independence.

Relevance: Vaccine risk monitoring, evaluation, and communications activities meaningfully address the needs of health professionals, policy makers, and the public.

Recommendation 1: A robust vaccine risk monitoring and evaluation office should develop and make public a strategic plan that encompasses input from health professionals, policy makers, and the public to ensure that the plan is scientifically sound, meets the needs and expectations of those who use the information, and articulates the office's role in monitoring, evaluating, and communicating vaccine risks.

---

[3] During the committee's deliberations, major changes were announced in the structure of CDC and its parent Department of Health and Human Services. To avoid possible confusion, the committee refers to ISO when describing the activities undertaken by that office before these reorganizations but to a federal vaccine risk monitoring and evaluation office for time periods after the start of those reorganizations.

Implementation steps:

1. Include a clear mission statement.
2. Establish a board of scientific counselors.
3. Develop a scientific agenda.
4. Develop mechanisms for bidirectional communication with health professionals and the public.
5. Outline action steps that will be taken in case of a public health emergency.

Relevance of vaccine risk monitoring and evaluation is dependent on a comprehensive strategic plan and clearly articulated mission. This plan ought to include clearly defined objectives and action steps, be publicly accessible, and incorporate meaningful input from diverse stakeholders— including health professionals, policy makers, and the public. Establishing a board of scientific counselors with deep scientific and communications expertise would enhance accountability, guide the strategic planning process, provide research advice, help ensure the independence of the vaccine risk monitoring and evaluation office, and support ongoing public engagement. Transparent communication of the scientific agenda and regular progress updates will help ensure that vaccine risk monitoring and evaluation activities remain aligned with public health priorities and needs and expectations of health professionals and the public.

Credibility: Health professionals, policy makers, and the public can rely on scientifically sound information and data analysis about vaccine risks.

Recommendation 2: A robust vaccine risk monitoring and evaluation office should be transparent and comprehensive in conducting and communicating its work in ways that are useful to health professionals, policy makers, and the public.

Implementation steps:

1. Focus on vaccine risk monitoring and evaluation, avoiding vaccine policymaking and promotion.
2. Develop a portfolio of publicly available information to explain systems and methodologic approaches, including data sources and system strengths and limitations, and priorities.
3. Ensure public availability of monitoring and evaluation protocols, including changes made during the data collection and analysis process and a justification for those changes.
4. Develop, disseminate, and evaluate accessible and easily understood plain language summaries of vaccine risk results.

5. Standardize risk reporting across communications and by risk groups, where available.

Credibility hinges on communicating vaccine risk information clearly, transparently, and comprehensively. This includes maintaining a clear distinction between vaccine risk evaluation and activities designed to increase use of vaccines to avoid perceived biases and conflicts of interest. To reinforce public trust, the office ought to regularly publish detailed explanations of its monitoring and evaluation systems, research methodologies, strengths, limitations, and key findings. Making these materials—including research protocols—publicly available, along with accessible, plain-language summaries and standardized risk reporting tailored for nonexpert audiences, will enhance transparency and significantly improve public understanding. The risk monitoring and evaluation experts ought to be consulted for technical accuracy, but other offices in CDC or HHS can use the risk information in policy determinations and communications.

Data Stewardship: Vaccine risk monitoring, evaluation, and communication activities are conducted with respect for the individuals whose data are used by protecting their privacy, using their data properly to address important questions about risks, and sharing the results.

Recommendation 3: A robust vaccine risk monitoring and evaluation office should be a good steward in the monitoring and evaluation processes by protecting the privacy of individuals and honoring their participation.

Implementation steps:

1. Protect personally identifiable information using appropriate standards.
2. Solicit input from researchers and the public about key elements of the research agenda.
3. Explore ways to make the data used in vaccine risk monitoring and evaluation more transparent, and where feasible and appropriate, available to external researchers.

Strong data stewardship is essential, requiring the ethical and secure handling of individual data. Rigorous data protection practices are necessary to safeguard participant privacy and ensure data confidentiality. Equally important is transparent communication about how data are collected and used and why. To promote scientific integrity and public trust, the office can work with its board of scientific counselors to explore secure, innovative methods for enabling controlled access to datasets by external researchers. This would support broader validation of findings, enhance transparency, and foster greater public confidence in vaccine risk monitoring.

Continuous Improvement and Innovation: Regular evaluation of vaccine risk monitoring, evaluation, and communication practices leads to adopting new methodologies and technologies with the capacity to address emerging questions about vaccine risks

> Recommendation 4: A robust vaccine risk monitoring and evaluation office should integrate continuous quality improvements into their strategic plan to strengthen their activities.

Implementation steps:

1. Develop metrics for evaluation in conjunction with strategic plan and advisors.
2. Maintain current data monitoring and evaluation systems and activities while incorporating advances in informatics, vaccinology, and epidemiological and statistical methods.
3. Use communication research, including in risk communication, to inform and assess their communications.

Continuous improvement and innovation are integral to the office's operational and strategic planning. This includes setting clear, measurable metrics for regular evaluation and systematically adopting advancements in vaccinology, epidemiology, statistical analysis, informatics, and communication practices. Regularly updating monitoring and evaluation systems and incorporating new technologies will help ensure that vaccine risk monitoring and evaluation remain responsive to evolving public health challenges. Additionally, investing in communication research will enhance the clarity, effectiveness, and impact of public messaging, strengthening audience engagement and understanding.

Independence: Vaccine risk monitoring, evaluation, and communication are free from undue internal or external influence.

> Recommendation 5: The Centers for Disease Control and Prevention (CDC) should protect the scientific independence of its vaccine risk monitoring office and provide the administrative support and financial resources to conduct these activities.

Implementation steps:

1. Keep the vaccine risk monitoring and evaluation office organizationally and administratively separated from units in CDC that carry out administrative or policymaking activities, such as promoting vaccination.
2. Increase awareness of the vaccine risk monitoring and evaluation work by clearly distinguishing risk information from vaccine policy content and that intended to increase immunization use.
3. Permit and encourage prompt publication of risk data.

Scientific independence is vital to the perceived impartiality, credibility, and effectiveness of vaccine risk data evaluation, communication, and contributions to practice. To protect its scientific integrity, the vaccine risk monitoring and evaluation office ought to remain organizationally and administratively separated from CDC units involved in vaccine promotion or policymaking. A distinct and clearly identifiable web presence for vaccine risk monitoring and evaluation and timely and unhindered publication of research findings—free from administrative interference—are essential for transparent, unbiased communication, and the delivery of scientifically rigorous information to the public. Scientific independence does not preclude consultation and collaboration with other CDC and government experts, but final decision making about monitoring and evaluation of vaccine risk information and the scientific content of risk communications needs to remain with this office.

Final Thoughts

Implementing these five recommendations would enhance the delivery of timely, trustworthy, and scientifically robust vaccine risk information and will require resources and the commitment of the CDC director. This, in turn, supports increased public confidence in vaccination programs, ultimately contributing to stronger public health outcomes and preparedness for future public health emergencies.

1

Introduction

On March 13, 2020, the Secretary of Health and Human Services (HHS) declared a nationwide public health emergency (PHE) due to the unfolding COVID pandemic (CDC, n.d.; NASEM, 2024). A key component of the response was the rapid development and deployment of new vaccines. While many organizations of the government were required to meet the challenges posed by the pandemic and the development of COVID vaccines, safety issues that might arise from their deployment fell in part to the Immunization Safety Office (ISO) in the Centers for Disease Control and Prevention (CDC). ISO plays a key role in monitoring and evaluating the risks of all vaccines, including COVID vaccines, once a decision has been reached that they can be administered to the public. ISO also oversees a set of complementary data collection and analysis systems, described later, crucial for updating vaccine recommendations.

The ISO requested that the National Academies of Sciences, Engineering, and Medicine convene an ad hoc committee of experts to evaluate its work on the safety of the COVID vaccines and recommend ways to improve all that it does. The task can be found in Box 1-1.

This chapter continues with a brief description of the history, structure, and function of vaccine safety assessment by ISO and others in the federal government, including during the COVID PHE. The chapter concludes with a set of guiding principles the committee used in framing its recommendations, followed by a brief description of the report structure and important terminology.

> **BOX 1-1**
> **Statement of Task**
>
> An ad hoc committee of the National Academies of Sciences, Engineering, and Medicine will evaluate the Centers for Disease Control and Prevention (CDC) Immunization Safety Office (ISO) systems, methods, and processes for monitoring COVID-19 vaccine safety during the U.S. COVID-19 vaccination program and provide recommendations for sustaining, maintaining, and strengthening CDC ISO current monitoring systems moving forward.
>
> Specifically, the committee will assess the statistical and epidemiological methods and processes employed to detect and evaluate potential safety problems with the U.S. COVID-19 vaccines; catalog the findings from safety monitoring including pertinent positive and negative findings; and evaluate CDC external communications about its safety monitoring systems, the findings of COVID-19 vaccine safety monitoring, and vaccination and clinical guidance recommendations to healthcare professionals, public health officials, and the public.[a]
>
> ---
>
> [a] Because ISO is not responsible for clinical guidance responsibilities, the committee evaluated the information ISO presented to those who do develop vaccine use recommendations. The committee did not evaluate the content of the clinical use guidelines.

VACCINE SAFETY ASSESSMENT

Vaccines have been an important public health tool for decades and were declared one of the 10 great public health achievements of the 20th century (CDC, 1999). They provide benefit to the vaccinated person and others. They prevent infections, protect against the most severe forms of disease, and prevent spread of infectious disease. The type and amount of protection depends on the target infection, specific vaccine, and recipient person or population.

Vaccines differ from pharmaceuticals in several important ways. While vaccines play a critical role in responding to immediate health threats, their greatest impact lies in the long-term prevention of infectious diseases across populations. Many vaccines are given to infants and children, so the decision to vaccinate is not theirs but that of their parent or guardian. Some vaccines are required or mandated for public school attendance, and some occupations can be subject to vaccine mandates as well.

Over the 20th century, vaccines became widely used and drove down the incidence of many once-common—and often deadly—infectious diseases in children. In recognition of their lifesaving impact, all 50 states adopted laws requiring one or more immunizations for school entry. As the appropriate use of vaccines was widely adopted, many communicable diseases were eliminated—such as smallpox—or dramatically reduced, including measles, mumps, whooping cough, and influenza. The threat of these serious and frequently life-threatening diseases faded (or appeared to fade) in the public's perception. Without an imminent threat of disease, fear of injury possibly related to vaccines led to a vaccine-related litigation environment (Blake, 2012; Grey, 2011).

Fearing that this increased liability would drive vaccine manufacturers out of the market, imperiling public health, Congress intervened in 1986 with the National Childhood Vaccine Injury Act (NCVIA) (Blake, 2012).[1] Recognizing that even the safest vaccine may produce some degree of harm in some individuals yet still serve the broader public, NCVIA limits liability for manufacturers (thus encouraging them to remain in the vaccine-making market) and ensures that injured persons have a mechanism for receiving compensation through the Vaccine Injury Compensation Program (Blake, 2012). The act also led to creating other important programs, such as the National Vaccine Program Office, Vaccine Adverse Event Reporting System (VAERS), and Vaccine Information Statements.

Questions about the safety of the COVID vaccines specifically arose for several reasons. Operation Warp Speed, a presidential initiative, led to the very rapid development and use of vaccines, two of which involved a novel technology, the mRNA platform. The vaccines were made available to the public initially through a legal provision known as "Emergency Use Authorization" (EUA) (see Box 1-2). Confusion about the EUA process made some hesitant to get vaccinated, due to the public misperception that the vaccines hadn't been rigorously assessed for risks. The safety profile of all COVID vaccines, including the mRNA vaccines, were studied in clinical trials as required by Food and Drug Administration (FDA), and risk monitoring and evaluation was launched by ISO staff as soon as vaccines were given to the public. However, public mistrust of government pandemic restrictions and policies began to spread, and trust in safety of the vaccines faltered (Funk et al., 2023).

CDC ISO

As described in Chapter 2, ISO's vaccine risk monitoring and evaluation involves staff and researchers, mostly from universities and health plans, who work under various contracts in support of various systems. These systems include the VSD, Clinical Immunization Safety Assessments,

---

[1] The National Childhood Vaccine Injury Act of 1986, Public Law 660, 99th Cong., October 14, 1986.

> **BOX 1-2**
> **Emergency Use Authorization (EUA)**
>
> The EUA mechanism is a legal provision allowing the Food and Drug Administration (FDA) to authorize not yet licensed medical products or unapproved uses of approved products during a public health emergency (PHE), as declared under Section 564 of the Federal Food, Drug, and Cosmetic Act (21 U.S.C. § 360bbb-3).
>
> **EUAs can be granted when**
>
> - A PHE is declared by the HHS Secretary,
> - FDA concludes that the product may be effective in diagnosing, treating, or preventing a serious or life-threatening disease,
> - The known and potential benefits outweigh known and potential risks, and
> - No adequate, approved, and available alternatives exist.
>
> **Key Differences from Standard Approval (BLA):**
>
> - Evidence Threshold: An EUA requires evidence from at least one well-conducted Phase 3 trial demonstrating that the product *may be effective* in preventing, diagnosing, or treating a serious or life-threatening disease and that the *known and potential benefits outweigh the known and potential risks.* For COVID vaccines, FDA required a median of at least 2 months of safety follow-up after completion of the primary series.
>   By contrast, a Biologics License Application (BLA) under Section 351 of the Public Health Service Act (42 U.S.C. § 262)[a] requires substantial evidence of effectiveness from adequate and well-controlled Phase 3 trials, longer-term safety data (typically 6 months or more of follow-up), and comprehensive submissions demonstrating manufacturing consistency, stability, pharmacovigilance planning, and compliance with labeling and facility standards.
> - Duration: EUAs are temporary and valid only during the declared emergency or until revoked. BLAs grant permanent licensure.
> - Postmarket Surveillance: EUA products are subject to thorough surveillance, such as through the Vaccine Adverse Event Reporting System (VAERS) and Vaccine Safety Datalink (VSD). Full licensure involves long-term postmarketing monitoring and periodic FDA inspections.
>
> ---
>
> [a] Public Health Service Act, Public Law 262, 42nd U.S. Congress, June 15, 2025.
> SOURCE: FDA, 2017.

VAERS (comanaged with FDA), V-safe, and a pregnancy registry. ISO data are an integral part of the deliberations of the Advisory Committee on Immunization Practices (ACIP), which makes vaccine recommendations, and FDA review of safety data related to postmarketing safety evaluations. See Figure 1-1 for the committee's understanding of how ISO's vaccine risk monitoring and evaluation moves from data collection to public communications, which will be described in more detail in Chapters 2 and 3.

For many years, vaccine risk monitoring and evaluation at CDC was the responsibility of the National Immunization Program (NIP). ISO was moved out of NIP in 2005 in response to concerns that the work of evaluating the risks from vaccines could not be done objectively if the staff were co-housed with the offices that promoted the use of vaccines (CDC, 2006). Between 2005 and 2010, ISO was in the CDC Office of the Chief Scientist, Office of the Director. In 2010, ISO was relocated to the CDC Division of Healthcare Quality Promotion (DHQP), National Center for Emerging Zoonotic Infectious Diseases (NCEZID), where it remains. NCEZID is organizationally distinct from the National Center for Immunization and Respiratory Diseases, with each reporting to the CDC director.

During the COVID PHE, monitoring and evaluating COVID vaccine risks postauthorization were conducted by ISO, contract staff, and other CDC staff on temporary detail, but due to temporary restructuring in response to the emergency declaration and creation of a government-wide response, these were carried out by the Vaccine Task Force (Gee, 2024). It was established at CDC; its incident manager reported to the CDC COVID agency response incident manager, who reported to the CDC director. ISO staff not deployed elsewhere performed data monitoring and evaluation work not as the "Immunization Safety Office" but within that task force (Su, 2024). Communications were coordinated through the Office of the Director, Department of Health and Human Services (HHS) Secretary, and White House (Jernigan, 2025). Chapter 2 discusses the data systems deployed to study the COVID vaccines, and Chapter 3 describes the communication processes.

See Box 1-3 for a list of ISO's official functions, as described in the Federal Register, which is consistent with the discussions the committee had with CDC in public sessions (Gee, 2024; Jernigan, 2025; Su, 2024). ISO does not have a dedicated website describing its structure, mission, and functions, although, as described in Chapter 3, voluminous CDC webpages address vaccine safety. For fiscal year (FY) 2020, before the public health declaration, the ISO budget was $22.5 million; staffing comprised 30 full-time employees (FTE) and eight contract staff. During the PHE (part of FY2020–part of FY2024), the range of annual funding, including supplemental funding, was $42–$114 million, and staffing levels were 37–47 FTE, with 122 contract staff. In FY2025, ISO annual funding is $51.5 million with staff of 43 FTE and 21 contract staff.[2] The funding derived from the NCEZID emerging infections program; NCIRD pandemic influenza program and Vaccines for Children Program; and targeted COVID funding.

Other Vaccine Safety Work in the Federal Government

Immunization work at CDC is but one piece of the larger federal government response to vaccine-preventable diseases generally and vaccine safety specifically (Gee et al., 2024) (see Table 1-1). Regulatory responsibility sits in FDA, which approves or authorizes vaccines and can require post-market surveillance of manufacturers. ISO and FDA scientists collaborate and communicate frequently (Gee, 2024), and VAERS, described in detail in Chapter 2, is the shared responsibility of FDA and CDC. Researchers at the Veterans Health Administration, Centers for Medicare & Medicaid Services, Indian Health Service, and Department of Defense conduct vaccine safety studies of importance to their mission; the populations of interest to them (e.g., veterans of all ages; elderly people and those with disabilities; and active duty military and some beneficiaries) are complementary to those studied in ISO's systems, as described in Chapter 2. Many other countries also have robust vaccine safety or pharmacovigilance units and publish data from those monitoring and evaluation systems, which complement or supplement the information generated in the United States.

COMMITTEE APPROACH TO THE STATEMENT OF TASK

The committee comprises expertise in administration of government public health, research and regulatory administration; pharmacoepidemiology; biostatistics; health literacy; health communication; clinical medicine and pharmacy; public health law; and public health practice (see Appendix A). It met numerous times in full and in small groups beginning in May 2024 and held five sessions open to the public. During three of these sessions, CDC presented information on the charge, the systems it uses to monitor and assess vaccine safety, and its communication process regarding vaccine safety. In addition, the committee held a public comment session at which 13 persons made 3-minute public comments in response to questions posed by the committee in advance:

- What criteria should CDC use when deciding how vaccine safety and potential harms from vaccines should be studied?
- How can CDC's research on vaccine safety and potential harms from vaccines be improved?

---

[2] Personal Communication, J. Gee, Centers for Disease Control and Prevention, August 5, 2025.

BOX 1-3
Key Functions of the Immunization Safety Office (ISO)

The ISO "assesses the safety of new and currently available vaccines received by children, adolescents and adults using a variety of strategies:

1. conducts ongoing surveillance for the timely detection of possible adverse events following immunization (AEFI) in collaboration with the Food and Drug Administration, through implementation and management of the Vaccine Adverse Event Reporting System, the national reporting system that acts as an early-warning system to detect health conditions that might be associated with an immunization;
2. coordinates, further develops, maintains and directs activities of the Vaccine Safety Datalink (VSD), a collaborative effort with integrated healthcare organizations able to perform rapid epidemiologic research on potential causality for AEFI using the VSD and other data sources, provide national estimates of incidence of AEFI, and determine background rates of health conditions;
3. leads the nation in developing biostatistical methods for research of AEFI using large linked databases and other data sources, and shares methods for use by other agencies and public and private entities;
4. conducts clinical research to identify causes of adverse events after immunization, specific populations susceptible to specific adverse events, and prevention strategies through the DHQP supported Clinical Immunization Safety Assessment network, a national network of medical research centers, and through other research efforts;
5. applies findings from epidemiologic and clinical studies to develop strategies for prevention of AEFI;
6. provides global consultation and leadership for the development, use, and interpretation of vaccine safety surveillance systems, and for the development of shared definitions of specific health outcomes through participation in the Brighton Collaboration and other international organizations
7. provides data for action to HHS, the Federal Advisory Committee on Immunization Practices (ACIP), the FDA's Vaccine and Related Biological Products Advisory Committee, Health Resources and Services Administration's Advisory Commission on Childhood Vaccines, and international collaborators including the WHO Global Advisory Committee on Vaccine Safety; and
8. provides timely, accurate communication and education to partners and the public on vaccine safety issues."

SOURCE: CDC, 2023.

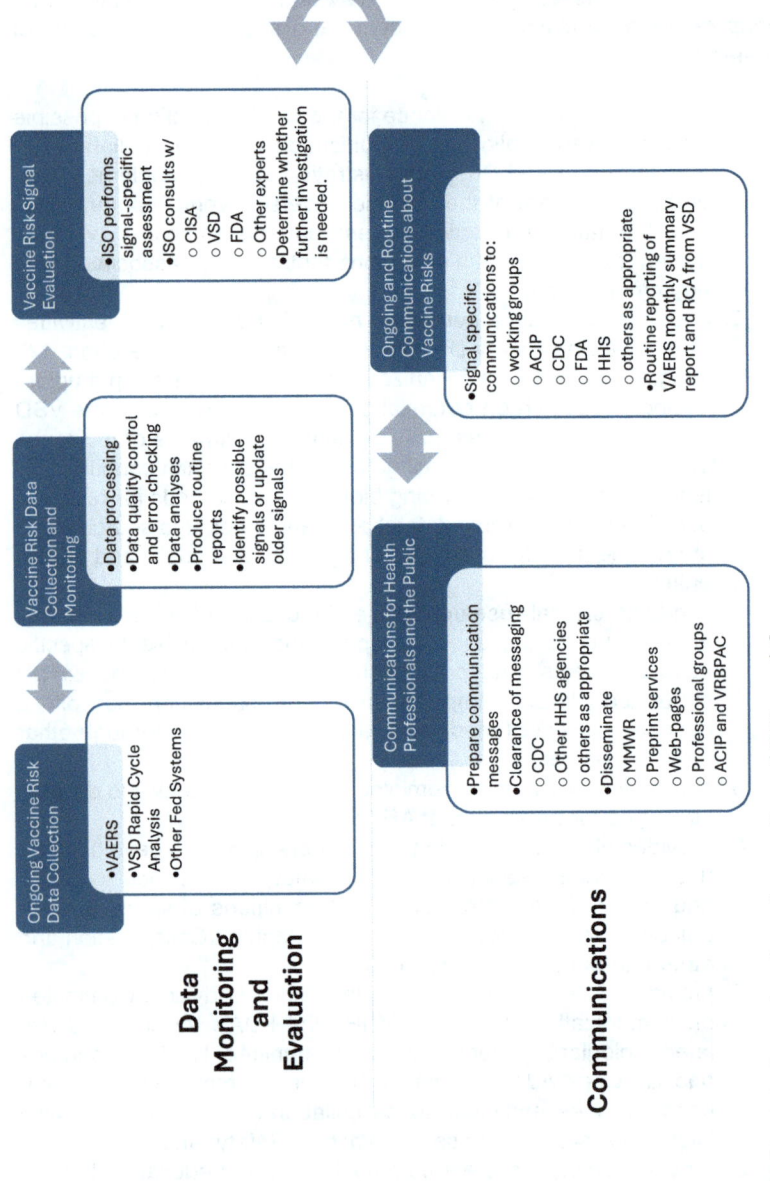

FIGURE 1-1 Committee's understanding of ISO workflow.

INTRODUCTION 23

TABLE 1-1 Vaccine Offices in the Department of Health and Human Services

Agency/ Department	Office	Function	Relevant Advisory Committee
CDC/HHS	ISO	Studies risks from vaccines	None
CDC/HHS	Immunization Services Division	Supports vaccine benefit assessment, promotion programs, and the coordination of national vaccine policy recommendations	ACIP
CBER/FDA/HHS	OVRR/OBP; Office of Biostatistics and Pharmacoepidemiology	Approves or authorizes vaccines for use; can mandate postmarketing studies by manufacturers; has joint responsibility for VAERS	Vaccines and Related Biologic Products Advisory Committee
OASH/HHS	National Vaccine Program, Office of Infectious Disease and HIV/AIDS Policy	Coordinates vaccine-related work across HHS (and the federal government)	National Vaccine Advisory Committee
HRSA	Division of Injury Compensation Programs	Along with Department of Justice, administers VICP and CICP	Advisory Committee on Childhood Vaccines

NOTES: Due to pending reorganization of HHS, this is accurate as of April 2025. ACIP = Advisory Committee on Immunization Practices; CBER = Center for Biologics Evaluation and Research; CDC = Centers for Disease Control and Prevention; CICP = countermeasure injury compensation program; FDA = Food and Drug Administration; HHS = Department of Health and Human Services; HRSA = Health Resources and Services Administration; ISO = Immunization Safety Office; OASH = Office of the Assistant Secretary for Health; OBP = Office of Biotechnology Products; OVRR = Overview of the Office of Vaccines Research and Review; VAERS = Vaccine Adverse Event Reporting System; VICP = Vaccine Injury Compensation Program.

- When should new findings or safety signals be shared with researchers, health professionals, and the public?
- How should CDC communicate new findings about vaccine safety or harms to the public?
- How can CDC improve Americans' confidence in the safety of vaccines though research and messaging?

See Box 1-4 for a summary of salient points.[3] Additionally, the committee held an open, public session with invited experts to discuss the challenges

---

[3] Appearance in this list does not mean the committee endorses the points made.

BOX 1-4
Salient Points from Public Comment

Monitoring and Evaluation

- CDC should improve vaccine safety research by adhering to its own protocols (such as proper proportional reporting ratio calculations) and funding further studies. Safety signals should be shared promptly, with full transparency. To rebuild public trust, CDC should support its claims with data and continue data collection even when findings challenge prior assumptions.
- Independent monitoring is crucial. Vaccine side effect reports should be collected and reviewed by a body separate from agencies responsible for promoting vaccination to ensure objectivity and public trust.
- The Vaccine Safety Datalink lacks public access, and public and independent researchers cannot easily access the data. Making it publicly available would enhance transparency and scientific scrutiny.
- CDC's ISO team should be commended for their efforts during the pandemic, but there is a clear need for a faster, more robust, and independent system to evaluate vaccine safety. This includes better funding, coordination, and a separation between risk assessment and risk management. Historically, a lack of conclusive science on vaccine reactions highlights the need for more research, including understanding biological mechanisms. While public health authorities and providers are generally well served, public needs remain unmet, contributing to distrust and polarization.
- Continued use of both active and passive surveillance systems (like Vaccine Adverse Event Reporting System, Vaccine Safety Datalink, and V-safe) is essential for capturing a wide range of vaccine safety data, aided by standardized definitions (e.g., from the Brighton Collaboration).

Communications

- While simple guidance may work for some, more detailed and nuanced recommendations are necessary for those seeking deeper understanding.
- Communication must be swift, comprehensive, and proactive, guiding health care providers in recognizing and responding to potential harms.
- While VAERS is a commonly cited, passive reporting system often criticized for its limitations, the United States also operates more robust vaccine safety tools that are far less known to the public.
- The United States has some of the most advanced systems in the world for monitoring vaccine safety, including tools that analyze electronic health records and provide expert clinical guidance. CDC also works with global collaborators to investigate potential risks such as myocarditis. Despite these efforts, public awareness remains low.
- CDC should do more to communicate the existence and value of its surveillance systems to build trust, promote transparency, and counter misinformation.
- When safety signals emerge, CDC must communicate rapidly and transparently, clarifying the distinction between evolving scientific data and policy decisions. This open, value-aware approach—tailored to different communities and partnered with trusted local leaders—can build trust, address ethical concerns, and respect varying perspectives on autonomy and public health.
- CDC should be clearer about both what it knows and what it doesn't know regarding vaccines to avoid misinformation and confusion. In addition, adverse events need more precise and transparent reporting; terms like "mild" or "moderate" can be misleading without concrete definitions. Acknowledging data gaps—rather than simply offering reassurances—can help maintain trust in CDC.
- Expressing benefits while downplaying risks of medical products erodes public trust. When official messaging contradicts personal experiences, it damages CDC's credibility.

SOURCE: Public Comment, October 11, 2024.

of studying and communicating vaccine risks with specific populations. See Appendix B for agendas of those meetings. Videos of all presentations are available on the project website (https://www.nationalacademies.org/our-work/review-of-cdc-covid-19-vaccine-safety-research-and-communications).

The committee commissioned a series of confidential key informant interviews (see Appendix C). It further oversaw the creation of case studies of COVID vaccine risks to illustrate the timeline of COVID vaccine risk information generation and communication (see Appendix D). It used the information from public meetings, key informant interviews, and case studies, in addition to CDC's website and published research, to inform its targeted analyses of ISO COVID vaccine risk monitoring and evaluation and communication.

The committee encountered challenges in information-gathering. As part of Project Clean Slate (CDC, 2024), CDC reorganized its website, making it difficult to identify webpages that were active during the PHE, the period of most of the committee's analysis. This was particularly important for assessing ISO's communications. Other information, such as the presentation on communications and information on ISO budgets, was provided much later than requested. The HHS pause in communications in early 2025 (Fink, 2025) resulted in no participation by ISO staff in the key informant interviews.

The committee considered several important issues about vaccine risk monitoring and evaluation out of scope for its task. Postmarketing safety requirements of vaccine manufacturers are the purview of FDA, and recommendations for vaccine use are the purview of the ACIP and the CDC director. While the committee discusses the implication of the administrative placement of ISO, conclusions and recommendations on that topic were not part of the statement of task. Finally, the committee was not asked to recommend a funding level for the office, although such an important office needs full financial support. Many of these issues are discussed as context for the committee's conclusions and recommendations. It reiterates that matters of vaccine use and clinical guidance recommendations are out of scope for ISO and therefore for this report.

The Committee's Guiding Principles

Reliable and impartial vaccine risk monitoring and evaluation are essential to health professionals, policy makers, and the public for informed decision making. ISO is a source of much of that information. Since all of ISO's products and communications are based on data collection and statistical analysis, the committee carefully studied the latest edition of Principles and Practices for a Federal Statistical Agency (NASEM, 2025) and adapted that for its recommendations. That report states that federal statistical agencies, which includes CDC's National Center for Health Statistics, and other designated offices "...provide objective and impartial information that informs policy makers and the public, they should not advocate policies or take partisan positions that would undercut public trust and credibility of the statistics they produce." The committee is not recommending that ISO be designated a Federal Statistical Agency, because that would exceed its remit and is not necessary to achieve the goals it has for vaccine risk monitoring and evaluation, which is that this office continues to merit the nation's trust. However, adherence to the principles that these agencies follow (see Chapter 4) provides a firm foundation for increased effectiveness and trust that are required for such an important mission:

- Relevance to Policy Issues and Society,
- Credibility Among Data Users and Stakeholders,
- Trust Among the Public and Data Subjects,
- Independence from Political and Other Undue External Influence, and
- Continuous Improvement and Innovation.

REPORT STRUCTURE AND TERMINOLOGY

Beginning in early 2025, HHS announced plans for a major reorganization. As best as possible, the committee uses the name of an office, agency, or department as it was during the period of review, that is, before the reorganization. Should an office change names or organizational placement, the committee intends that its statements, including conclusions and recommendations, still apply to the relevant office.

In this report, the committee chooses to use "vaccine risk" to describe serious, untoward effects of vaccines. This would not include more minor, common, and predictable side effects, such as time-limited fever, malaise, arthralgia, and myalgia, although ISO systems such as VAERS capture these. Additionally, although the committee recognizes that some of ISO's work is hypothesis-driven research, ISO also performs routine monitoring. Despite ISO's name, the committee uses "vaccine risk monitoring and evaluation" to describe ISO's work instead of "immunization safety." To some, "safety" reflects a balance of risks and benefits, and to others, it implies 100 percent safe or risk free. Furthermore, safety concerns include things like manufacturing errors or contaminations, which are FDA regulatory concerns.

The report contains a summary, appendixes, and four chapters: this introductory Chapter 1, Chapter 2 on ISO's data monitoring and evaluation programs, Chapter 3 on ISO communications, and Chapter 4, which offers three conclusions and five recommendations. Three appendixes include substantive information that the committee used as part of its analysis: the independently authored report from confidential key informant interviews (Appendix C), the committee-directed case studies (Appendix D), and a catalog of ISO COVID vaccine publications (Appendix E).

REFERENCES

Blake, V. 2012. The National Childhood Vaccine Injury Act and the Supreme Court's interpretation. *AMA Journal of Ethics* 14(1):31–34. https://doi.org/10.1001/virtualmentor.2012.14.1.hlaw1-1201

CDC (Centers for Disease Control and Prevention). n.d. *CDC Museum COVID-19 Timeline.* https://www.cdc.gov/museum/timeline/covid19.html#Early-2020 (accessed April 16, 2025).

CDC. 1999. *Ten great public health achievements—United States, 1900–1999.* Washington, DC: Centers for Disease Control and Prevention.

CDC. 2006. *Advisory Committee on Immunization Practices Record of the Proceedings.* Washington, DC: Centers for Disease Control and Prevention. https:/www.cdc.gov/vaccines/acip/meetings/downloads/min-archive/min-2006-06-508.pdf (archived on March 8, 2021 using the Wayback Machine: https://web.archive.org/web/20210308230331).

CDC. 2023. *Reorganization of the National Center for Emerging and Zoonotic Infectious Diseases.* https://www.federalregister.gov/documents/2023/07/12/2023-14704/reorganization-of-the-national-center-for-emerging-and-zoonotic-infectious-diseases (accessed August 26, 2025).

CDC. 2024. *CDC.Gov CleanSlate and relaunch URL mappings.* https://data.cdc.gov/dataset/CDC-gov-CleanSlate-and-Relaunch-URL-Mappings/vyry-2yfg/about_data (accessed July 29, 2025).

FDA (Food and Drug Administration). 2017. *Emergency Use Authorization of Medical Products and Related Authorities.* Washington, DC: Department of Health and Human Services.

Fink, D. A. 2025. *Immediate pause on issuing documents and public communications—ACTION.* Washington, DC: Department of Health and Human Services.

Funk, C., A. Tyson, B. Kennedy, and P. Giancarlo. 2023. *Americans' largely positive views of childhood vaccines hold steady.* Washington, DC: Pew Research Center.

Gee, J. 2024. CDC response to vaccine safety needs for the U.S. COVID-19 vaccination program—an overview of vaccine safety systems. Presentation to the Committee to Review the Centers for Disease Control and Prevention's (CDC) COVID-19 Vaccine Safety Research and Communications, Washington, DC, August 7.

Gee, J., T. T. Shimabukuro, J. R. Su, D. Shay, M. Ryan, S. V. Basavaraju, K. R. Broder, M. Clark, C. B. Creech, and F. Cunningham. 2024. Overview of U.S. COVID-19 vaccine safety surveillance systems. *Vaccine* 42:125748.

Grey, B. J. 2011. The plague of causation in the national childhood vaccine injury act. *Harvard Journal on Legislation* 48:343.

Jernigan, D. 2025. CDC COVID-19 vaccine safety risk communications. Presentation to the Committee to Review the Centers for Disease Control and Prevention's (CDC) COVID-19 Vaccine Safety Research and Communications, January 10. Washington, DC.

NASEM (National Academies of Sciences, Engineering, and Medicine). 2024. *Evidence review of the adverse effects of COVID-19 vaccination and intramuscular vaccine administration.* Washington, DC: The National Academies Press.

NASEM. 2025. *Principles and practices for a federal statistical agency: Eighth edition.* Washington, DC: The National Academies Press.

Su, J. R. 2024. U.S. Centers for Disease Control and Prevention COVID-19 vaccine safety monitoring from December 2020–May 2023. Presentation to the Committee to Review the Centers for Disease Control and Prevention's (CDC) COVID-19 Vaccine Safety Research and Communications, Washington, DC, June 24, 2024.

2

Data Monitoring and Evaluation

During the COVID public health emergency (PHE), the Centers for Disease Control and Prevention (CDC) Immunization Safety Office (ISO) played a critical role in monitoring and evaluating the safety of vaccines administered under unprecedented conditions. Leveraging existing surveillance systems and rapidly scaling new monitoring platforms, ISO implemented a comprehensive monitoring and evaluation framework (Klein et al., 2021; Shimabukuro et al., 2021a). This chapter outlines ISO's data-driven efforts to detect, assess, and respond to potential safety concerns in real time, highlighting the integration of information from traditional systems, like the Vaccine Adverse Event Reporting System (VAERS) and Vaccine Safety Datalink (VSD), with enhanced tools, such as V-safe and the Clinical Immunization Safety Assessment (CISA) Project.

The safety monitoring infrastructure described in this report informed public health policy makers throughout the COVID vaccination campaign. Early identification of signals of potential adverse events (AEs), such as thrombosis with thrombocytopenia syndrome (TTS), myocarditis, and Guillain-Barré syndrome (GBS), allowed for timely clinical guidance, reduced preventable morbidity, and informed risk–benefit assessments for distinct populations (Greinacher et al., 2021; Montgomery et al., 2021; See et al., 2021). Using a range of methods—from passive surveillance in VAERS to active, population-based analyses of VSD—policy makers and scientists were able to triangulate signals, confirm or refute potential associations, and refine vaccination recommendations in real time (McNeil et al., 2014). While comprehensive and effective monitoring efforts were evident, the complex nature of the data from the evaluation programs sometimes challenged the ability to clearly and succinctly communicate findings to the public and health care providers (HCPs), limiting the potential to do even greater good for the public's health (Salmon et al., 2021).

Vaccine safety research spans a spectrum of study designs that vary in their ability to detect different categories of AEs. Randomized controlled trials and early-phase studies are optimized to reveal common, often immunologically mediated reactogenic events that occur within hours to days (Baden et al., 2021; Polack et al., 2020); however, their modest sample sizes (typically ≤50,000) lack the statistical power to uncover events with incidence below ~1 per 10,000 doses (Black et al., 2009). Large postauthorization observational designs—self-controlled case series, cohort analyses, and population-level data linkage studies—are therefore essential for estimating the incidence of less-common outcomes (1 per 10,000–100,000), such as myocarditis or anaphylaxis (Klein et al., 2021; Petersen et al., 2016). VSD was designed to perform these large postauthorization studies; however, extremely rare events (<1 per 100,000), like TTS or GBS, require even broader, often multinational data pools, case-control networks, and rapid cycle analyses (RCAs) of health care databases that aggregate tens of millions of vaccinated person-years to achieve adequate signal-to-noise ratios (Faksova et al., 2024). Finally, mechanistic bench-to-bedside investigations, although infrequently funded, are critical to elucidate causal pathways once epidemiologic associations are flagged (Das, 2023; Moro et al., 2019). Mechanistic investigations are rare, so the biology underlying most serious, vaccine-associated AEs remains unknown.

An essential component of these vaccine safety evaluations was the ongoing review and oversight provided by the Advisory Committee on Immunization Practices (ACIP) and its COVID-19 Vaccines Safety Technical (VaST) Work Group. Building on foundational vaccine safety studies ranging from preclinical trials to Phase 4 postauthorization evaluations, ACIP and VaST functioned as critical technical groups tasked with independently reviewing data generated by ISO's postauthorization surveillance systems. VaST regularly assessed emerging safety signals, interpreted complex data from diverse surveillance mechanisms, and communicated these findings during ACIP meetings (Markowitz et al., 2024). The goal of these deliberations was to inform timely updates to vaccine recommendations to provide alignment with the latest safety data and public health needs.

Beyond the immediate pandemic context, the integrated approach to vaccine safety monitoring exemplified by ISO, ACIP, and VaST underscores the importance of a multilayered surveillance program with coordinated and complementary strategies for detecting and addressing both common and extremely rare AEs. The continuous feedback loop—emerging signals prompting further epidemiologic studies and expert clinical consultation—ensures that vaccine policy decisions remain evidence based and responsive to evolving real-world conditions. Ultimately, the goal of this adaptive, science-driven safety network is to provide a foundation for sustained improvements in vaccine safety oversight and rapid global health responses moving forward.

ISO MONITORING AND EVALUATION/ASSESSMENT SYSTEMS

To monitor the safety of COVID vaccines during the PHE, CDC leveraged a coordinated network of complementary surveillance systems. Each system played a distinct role within the broader safety infrastructure—ranging from early signal detection to in-depth clinical evaluation. In this report, we use "signal detection" to refer to identifying a potential vaccine safety concern based on early surveillance data—typically in passive or high-throughput systems, such as RCAs done by VSD. "Signal evaluation" encompasses the follow-up activities used to further characterize the strength, direction, and potential causal nature of an observed association, including what VSD reports traditionally describe as signal refinement and evaluation. While we recognize that these phases can be conceptually distinct, they often occur along a continuum and are treated as part of an integrated process for assessing vaccine safety. VAERS served as the primary tool for signal detection, flagging potential AEs through standardized analyses of spontaneous reports from throughout the United States. VSD was used for signal detection through standardized RCAs and data-mining approaches, like TreeScan, but also the primary tool for population-based signal evaluation using electronic health records from a set of 11 large, integrated health care systems.[1] In addition to consultative activities, the CISA Project provided technical expertise and clinical guidance to evaluate rare or complex cases that required specialized review. CDC also launched V-safe, a new smartphone-based, active-surveillance platform designed to rapidly collect self-reported, postvaccination health experiences, particularly common local and systemic reactions, supporting a registry of vaccinated individuals. To monitor outcomes among pregnant individuals, the V-safe COVID-19 Vaccine Pregnancy Registry was established as a targeted follow-up system to track maternal and infant outcomes over time. Together, these systems formed a multilayered approach to identifying, assessing, and responding to vaccine safety concerns in near real time.

---

[1] VSD has 13 participating sites; 11 provide data, and the remaining two offer subject-matter expertise.

VAERS

VAERS is a national passive surveillance program comanaged by CDC and the Food and Drug Administration (FDA). Established in 1990, VAERS aims to detect early signals of possible vaccine-related AEs (CDC, 2024a). HCPs and vaccine manufacturers are legally mandated to report specific postvaccination events, and patients or caregivers may also submit reports. Although these data are crucial for generating hypotheses on vaccine safety concerns, they are usually insufficient to determine causality (Gee et al., 2024). VAERS may provide reasonable certainty for events such as anaphylaxis within minutes of administration (Shimabukuro et al., 2021a) or previously unrecognized diseases (such as TTS) shortly after vaccination (Shay et al., 2021). However, the determination of rates of AEs attributable to vaccines needs to be performed in data systems that do not rely on selective passive reporting. In addition, for most other events, data collected through active-surveillance systems and controlled epidemiological designs are required to help establish a causal relationship between a vaccine and an AE.

During the PHE, VAERS played a particularly prominent role in safety monitoring. VAERS data were reviewed in near real time. The heightened public interest in COVID vaccine safety led to increased transparency around VAERS data, with CDC and FDA issuing frequent public communications, updating online dashboards, and providing summaries of key findings. When signals like myocarditis and TTS were identified, more detailed investigations were done using both VAERS and VSD and sometimes led to revised vaccination guidance (Gargano et al., 2021; Shay et al., 2021).

VAERS collects and codes all spontaneously reported AEs among the vaccinated. Prespecified AEs of special interest (AESI) were selected for enhanced safety monitoring based on biological plausibility, previous vaccine safety experience, and theoretical concerns related to COVID vaccines. By protocol, medical records and autopsies were requested for AESIs and all serious events (e.g., death) for further clinical investigation. In addition to the prespecified AEs, symptoms identified during this enhanced surveillance were added to VAERS as AESIs only for COVID vaccines (Oliver et al., 2020).

VAERS, as a passive surveillance system, is inherently limited by underreporting, variability in data completeness, and differential reporting across time and populations (Shimabukuro et al., 2015; Varricchio et al., 2004). While some reports may be incomplete or lack medical confirmation, outright fabrication is believed to be rare (CDC, 2024a; HHS, 2024). A more common limitation is preferential or stimulated reporting—where known or suspected AEs are more likely to be reported in the context of a new vaccine rollout, media attention, or scientific publications. In addition, it lacks control groups of nonvaccinated persons, making it difficult to assess whether an AE is simply consistent with background rates (Varricchio et al., 2004). However, within the broader vaccine safety ecosystem, VAERS serves a vital function in the earliest stages of monitoring by highlighting patterns that warrant deeper study (Shimabukuro et al., 2015).

The VAERS experience during the COVID pandemic underscores its adaptability and value. The required reporting of vaccine denominator information (doses administered), expanded reporting mandates, and real-time analytical methods all contributed to more robust safety surveillance (Zou et al., 2022). While VAERS alone cannot establish causation, its ability to detect safety signals—especially when integrated with other active-surveillance platforms that can further evaluate them—proved critical for rapidly identifying potential concerns informing further investigation and evidence-based policy (Gargano et al., 2021).

VAERS summary-level data are publicly downloadable through CDC WONDER, but case-level narratives, medical records, and personally identifiable information are protected. Investigators seeking detailed, deidentified case-level datasets must submit a formal data request to CDC/FDA, sign a data-use agreement (DUA), and obtain Institutional Review Board (IRB) or other ethics approval. Aggregate surveillance tables and weekly data-mining outputs are posted on the CDC VAERS website and updated dashboards.

Analysis of VAERS data requires methodology that accounts for spontaneous reporting. For example, VAERS investigators have used an estimate called the "proportional reporting ratio" (PRR) to detect AEs that occur more frequently than expected after a vaccine. For COVID vaccines, this involves comparing the proportion of a specific AE among all reported AEs to the proportion of that same AE among AEs reported for other vaccines. If the AE occurs more often with the COVID vaccine, it may signal a safety concern. The PRR can be further analyzed by factors like age group, AE severity, and vaccine type. A potential safety signal is typically defined as a PRR of 2 or higher, a chi-squared value of at least 4 (indicating that it is unlikely to be due to chance), and at least three reports of the AE for that vaccine (Shimabukuro et al., 2015). FDA uses a related method—Empirical Bayesian data mining—to identify signals when the lower bound of the 95 percent confidence interval of the empirical Bayes geometric mean exceeds a predefined threshold. However, both CDC and FDA interpreted these methods with caution during the COVID response. The utility of PRR was limited because of enhanced and widespread reporting for COVID vaccines, which made historical comparisons less meaningful. As a result, most safety assessments relied on reported rates of specific AEs—calculated as the number of reports per doses administered—rather than PRR (Sakaeda et al., 2013). This approach was newly possible due to valuable national tracking of administration. Before the pandemic, crude rates of AEs could be only approximated based on estimated doses of vaccines administered. However, the federal government instituted additional reporting requirements for COVID vaccines (CDC, 2023; Gee et al., 2021). Tracking for each dose administered included information on recipient age and sex, manufacturer, and dose number (CDC, 2024b; Klein et al., 2021). This enabled precise denominators and allowed for calculating reported rates of AESIs—that is, the number of reported events per number of vaccine doses administered over a specified risk window (e.g., 1 or 21 days) (Shimabukuro et al., 2021a). These reported rates could be stratified by specific vaccine, age, and sex and compared to expectations based on published background rates. Since reporting to VAERS is not complete, reported rates would usually be expected to be less than background rates. Nevertheless, if a statistical signal emerged—via PRR, empirical Bayesian data mining, or observed rates approaching or exceeding background—a clinical review would be triggered that considered seriousness, biological plausibility, and consistency with a known clinical syndrome (Shimabukuro et al., 2015). Data mining and review of serious events and AESIs occurred daily at ISO (Gee et al., 2024). The VAERs team met weekly to review tables and clinical reports and discuss signals. Cumulative tabulations, including frequency of AEs and relative proportions by seriousness, sex, and age, were publicly available weekly (to CDC WONDER,[2] HHS, and Epi-X[3]). In parallel, ISO and FDA staff held weekly or ad hoc coordination meetings to review new VAERS data and emerging safety concerns (Anderson, 2020).

VSD

VSD is a collaborative project between CDC and 13 large, integrated U.S. health care organizations. It is the ISO's flagship active-surveillance platform, absorbing the majority of ISO's analytic resources (McNeil et al., 2014). Established in 1990, VSD uses electronic health records (EHRs) and health care use administrative data (claims) from millions of individuals receiving routine health care within participating systems and has grown from about 6 million covered members at launch to more than 12 million (CDC, 2024c; Chen et al., 1997; Wallace et al., 2022). Of the 13 sites, 11 provide EHR data. This design allows for more robust analyses than passive reporting systems because it includes well-defined population denominators, unvaccinated control populations, longitudinal patient data, and

---

[2] Centers for Disease Control and Prevention Wide-ranging Online Data for Epidemiologic Research (CDC WONDER) is an online system that provides access to a broad array of public health information and datasets.

[3] Epidemic Information Exchange (EPI-X) is CDC's secure, web-based communication system for sharing preliminary health surveillance and outbreak information with public health officials.

the capacity to perform population-based comparative studies (McNeil et al., 2014; Wallace et al., 2022). VSD's common data model substantially overlaps with that used by the FDA-funded Sentinel Initiative, and several partner sites contribute data to both programs, facilitating shared analytic code and cross-network validation (FDA, 2017). VSD researchers commonly use epidemiological approaches, including RCA and self-controlled risk interval designs, to detect and evaluate potential vaccine-related safety signals in near real time. Specifically, RCA involves weekly sequential hypothesis testing—often employing maximized sequential probability ratio tests—to compare observed AE counts against expected baselines, enabling VSD to flag potential safety signals within weeks of vaccine administration (Davis, 2013).

During the PHE, VSD expanded its analytical frequency and leveraged its comprehensive electronic data to provide timely assessments of COVID vaccines (CDC, 2024c; Klein, 2021). This included near-real-time monitoring of AESIs—such as myocarditis, TTS, and other events flagged by passive systems—to characterize incidence rates, identify potential risk factors (e.g., age, sex, comorbidities), and compare rates with background rates in unvaccinated or prepandemic populations (Klein, 2021). The close integration of EHR and administrative claims data enabled rapid turnaround for signal detection and evaluation, contributing to prompt public health guidance (CDC, 2024c). While VSD's focused, population-based approach offers advantages in assessing causality and absolute risks, it is concentrated within certain health care systems, does not capture all geographic or demographic groups (McNeil et al., 2014). Nevertheless, its ability to provide active surveillance at scale and rigorous, real-time data analyses has been particularly valuable during the heightened vaccine safety monitoring requirements of the pandemic (CDC, 2024c).

Because VSD relies on protected EHR and insurance-claims data from participating health systems, individual-level datasets remain behind secure firewalls at each site. External researchers may collaborate through vetted protocol proposals reviewed by the VSD Research Committee; approved projects operate under data-sharing agreements, HIPAA waivers, and IRB approvals, with analyses executed on site and only aggregate results released. Public-facing safety updates and peer-reviewed manuscripts are posted on the CDC VSD webpage.

CISA

CISA is a national network of vaccine safety experts coordinated by CDC and funded through collaborative agreements with academic medical centers. Established in 2001, CISA was designed to provide specialized clinical consultation on complex or severe AEs following immunization (CDC,

2024d). By drawing on multidisciplinary expertise—infectious disease specialists, immunologists, allergists, and epidemiologists—CISA enhances CDC's capacity to investigate rare, high-impact vaccine safety signals that may not be fully understood through passive or broad-based active surveillance alone (e.g., VAERS or VSD) (Williams et al., 2011).

Throughout its history, CISA has fulfilled two core functions. First, it provides individualized clinical consultations, offering expert, case-by-case evaluations for HCPs managing unusual or severe postvaccination events (Williams et al., 2011). These consultations often involve comprehensive medical-record reviews, direct communication with treating clinicians, and, when necessary, advanced diagnostic testing. Second, CISA conducts mechanistic and observational research, including small cohort studies, case-control analyses, and mechanistic investigations, to explore the biological pathways that may underlie rare AEs following immunization (Williams et al., 2011). During the COVID PHE, these functions were adapted and intensified to support rapid, evidence-based responses to emerging vaccine safety concerns (CDC, 2024d).

During the PHE, CISA rapidly pivoted to address emerging signals tied to novel COVID vaccines. For example, it engaged in detailed case series study of TTS and cerebral venous sinus thrombosis (MacNeil et al., 2021). This single mechanistic study found no evidence that polyethylene glycol (a vaccine component) was responsible for anaphylaxis observed with several COVID vaccines (Zhou et al., 2023). Data collection and dissemination accelerated in response to real-time clinical demands: CISA expanded its consultation footprint, offered expedited reviews, and collaborated more intensively with other CDC surveillance systems (such as V-safe and VAERS) to synthesize findings (CDC, 2024d). These adaptations ensured that frontline clinicians and policy makers received timely, evidence-based guidance on preventing, identifying, and managing severe postvaccination events in an evolving pandemic landscape.

CISA consultation records and mechanistic-study data contain identifiable clinical details and therefore are not publicly released. Qualified investigators can access deidentified analytic files or collaborate on joint analyses after submitting a proposal to the CISA executive committee and obtaining IRB clearance and a CDC DUA. Summaries of consultation trends and key study findings are published in CDC reports, ACIP slide decks, and peer-reviewed journals.

V-safe

V-safe was developed and funded by Oracle Health Services and CDC to monitor vaccine safety in near real time (CDC, 2024e; Myers et al., 2023). Launched in December 2020 specifically to track AEs following

COVID vaccination, V-safe was designed to complement existing passive (e.g., VAERS) and active (e.g., VSD) surveillance systems by capturing self-reported health information directly from vaccine recipients. The system leverages text messaging and secure Web-based surveys to collect data on prespecified common postvaccination symptoms (e.g., fever, injection-site reactions) and more serious events that warrant medical attention (Gee et al., 2021; Myers et al., 2023).

In addition to prespecified items, an open-ended prompt collects free-text comments. Natural language inference models can be used to identify patterns (e.g., identifying "missed period" and "PMS" as menstrual irregularities) not solicited as prespecified symptoms. Upon enrollment, vaccinated individuals receive regular check-ins—initially daily, then transitioning to weekly—to document any new or ongoing symptoms (Hause et al., 2022a). This approach generates a robust stream of data that can be analyzed rapidly for emerging safety signals. Proportions of participants reporting local and systemic reactions and health impacts are tabulated by age, sex and severity. Through unique user links, V-safe also tailors reminders about subsequent vaccine doses, thus maintaining participant engagement throughout a multidose regimen. While originally introduced to serve as a rapid-response tool during the height of the PHE, V-safe underwent incremental refinements to accommodate booster doses, track pediatric vaccination, and expand the types of outcomes assessed. In particular, the COVID-19 Vaccine Pregnancy Registry is an expansion of V-safe (CDC, 2024f). These enhancements also included more targeted symptom queries (e.g., specific rare AEs) and refined protocols for transferring serious or urgent reports into more intensive follow-up systems, like the VAERS or the CISA project. As a result of these iterative improvements, V-safe evolved into one of CDC's largest and most frequently used active-surveillance platforms (CDC, 2024e; Gee, 2024; Gee et al., 2021).

While V-safe played a crucial role in capturing high-volume, near-real-time data on expected, nonserious postvaccination symptoms (e.g., fatigue, injection-site pain), it was less effective for serious AEs. Its structure—requiring smartphone access and voluntary, ongoing survey participation—limits detection of severe AEs, especially those that are incapacitating (Gee et al., 2021, 2024). Available publications suggest V-safe contributed primarily reactogenicity data rather than AE signals, and few known AESIs appear to have originated from V-safe and triggered follow-up in other systems (Gee et al., 2024; Hause et al., 2022a).

Designed, built, and supported under a donation agreement with Oracle Health Services and the Department of Health and Human Services, V-safe's public–private partnership raises important sustainability considerations: once emergency-phase federal funding ends, continued functionality will depend on long-term governance, dedicated appropriations, and ongoing collaboration with private-sector technology partners (Shimabukuro, 2023b).

Raw V-safe responses include contact information and protected health data and are stored on secure CDC servers. Researchers may request deidentified datasets through a formal application process requiring a CDC DUA, evidence of IRB approval, and data-security documentation. High-level statistics on local/systemic reactions, health-impact measures, and participation metrics are released periodically via the CDC V-safe dashboard and in MMWR safety summaries.

COVID-19 Vaccine Pregnancy Registry

CDC established the COVID-19 Vaccine Pregnancy Registry in December 2020, coinciding with the initial rollout of COVID vaccines under Emergency Use Authorization (EUA). Recognizing the exclusion of pregnant individuals from early-phase clinical trials, the registry was developed as a targeted postauthorization surveillance mechanism to actively collect safety data in this high-priority population. It was one of several initiatives supported under the authorities of the Public Readiness and Emergency Preparedness (PREP) Act and COVID vaccine EUA framework, which enabled expedited deployment of safety monitoring infrastructure during the PHE (CDC, 2024f; Gee et al., 2024; Moro et al., 2021).

The registry leveraged V-safe as a primary mechanism for enrollment. Individuals who received a COVID vaccine and reported their pregnancy status through V-safe were contacted and invited to participate. Approximately 23,000 people who reported receiving a COVID vaccine during pregnancy—or within 30 days before conception—were enrolled between December 2020 and June 2021, and about 85 percent consented to medical-record review, yielding a large, well-documented cohort for analyses of maternal and infant outcomes (Madni et al., 2024). This registry functioned as a critical component of the broader postauthorization safety surveillance system coordinated by CDC and FDA to ensure continuous monitoring under EUA. Upon consent, participants were followed prospectively through pregnancy and postpartum. Data collection included self-reported health information, pregnancy outcomes (e.g., spontaneous abortion, stillbirth, gestational age at delivery), and infant outcomes through the first few months. When feasible, registry participation also involved medical-record abstraction to validate outcomes.

During the PHE, the registry protocol was updated to reflect changes in vaccine availability (such as bivalent booster rollout), evolving clinical guidance (timing of vaccination during pregnancy), and emerging questions about maternal–fetal antibody transfer and neonatal protection. These updates were supported by the CARES Act, which enabled rapid scaling of data-collection infrastructure and digital tools through enhanced federal investment. The PREP Act also authorized emergency measures, including liability protections for vaccine administrators and manufacturers, facilitating operational flexibility for surveillance activities (Shimabukuro et al., 2021b).

Primary data sources for the registry included V-safe reports, structured participant surveys, and medical-record reviews. In select cases, linkage to other CDC-managed surveillance systems, such as the National Vital Statistics System, was conducted to enhance outcome verification (CDC, 2024f; Myers et al., 2023).

Due to the identifiable health information and sensitive nature of pregnancy-related data, access to individual-level registry data is restricted. Researchers and public health partners may request deidentified datasets or analytic summaries through formal CDC DUAs and IRB approvals. Public-facing summaries, including key outcome statistics and updated methodological details, are made available via the CDC COVID-19 Vaccine Pregnancy Registry webpage.

MAJOR METHODOLOGIC STRENGTHS/ LIMITATIONS OF FINDINGS/SAFETY ASSESSMENTS FROM EACH OF THE MAJOR SYSTEMS

The strengths and limitations of each vaccine safety surveillance system reflect their underlying design and intended role within the broader monitoring framework. Passive systems are best suited for early signal detection and hypothesis generation, offering national reach and transparency but limited by selection, underreporting, and reporting biases. Active-surveillance systems enable more robust, population-based analyses using EHRs with prospectively recorded information but operate within a defined health care network and require longer timelines for complex evaluations. CISA offered expert case reviews and mechanistic insights, particularly for complex or rare events. V-safe provided rapid, participant-reported data on reactogenicity and short-term outcomes but lacked medical validation. Its pregnancy registry allowed longitudinal tracking of vaccine safety during pregnancy. Like VAERS, V-safe does not include unvaccinated persons that can be used for comparisons. Together, these systems formed a complementary network—each with unique contributions but also important constraints that shaped how and when safety questions could be answered. Table 2-1 presents a comparative snapshot of each platform's principal advantages and constraints1.

In parallel, a range of other vaccine safety systems—operated by FDA, the Department of Veterans Affairs, the Indian Health Service, CMS,

TABLE 2-1 Key Strengths and Limitations of CDC COVID Vaccine Safety Surveillance Systems

Surveillance System	Strengths	Limitations	Use During COVID
VAERS*	National coverage and availability Early signal detection capability Captures broad range of AEs Publicly accessible data Event rates can be estimated when national statistics on vaccination rates are tracked	Variability in data completeness No control group; cannot establish causality Stimulated reporting due to media or public attention can inflate reports for certain events, potentially leading to false signals. Difficult to estimate accurate rates for vaccinations without denominator information (i.e., number vaccinated) Passive reporting leads to underreporting and underestimation of rates Limited geographic and demographic diversity (primarily large integrated health care systems representing an insured population) Longer timelines needed for complex evaluations	Over 1 million reports related to vaccines submitted by March 2022; prioritized review of AESIs and serious events under EUA
VSD	Active surveillance with defined denominators Population-based analyses using EHR data coupled with ability to perform medical-record review Prospective recording of vaccine and AEs reduces selection biases Ability to conduct near-real-time signal evaluation	Delays in data availability due to EHR and claims processing and validation procedures	RCA used to monitor ~23 AESIs weekly; studies included millions of vaccinated individuals (e.g., 6.2 million in myocarditis study)

CISA Project	Supports comparative risk analyses and adjustment for potential confounders	Limited numbers for subgroup analyses of serious, rare AEs	Provided expert input on emerging AESIs (e.g., myocarditis); developed clinical guidance and supported case adjudication
	Gathering information for expert clinical consultation for complex or rare AEs	Small case numbers limits generalizability and reach	
	In-depth chart reviews and diagnostic investigations	Case evaluations sometimes include confounding factors, like SARS-CoV-2 co-infection	
	Supports mechanistic research into vaccine-related events	Mechanistic studies, being resource intensive, are rarely performed	
V-safe#	Rapid, participant-reported data collection	Self-reported data without medical-record validation	Over 10 million enrollees in first year; enabled daily symptom monitoring; linked to pregnancy registry for follow-up
	Focus on common postvaccination symptoms	Outcomes dependent on participant retention and data completeness	
	Captures near-real-time data on newly vaccinated individuals	Potential selection bias (voluntary enrollment)	
	Adaptive system with evolving questionnaires	Limited capacity to detect rare or serious AEs due to reliance on self-enrollment and active survey response; may underrepresent severely ill individuals	
		No unvaccinated persons for comparison	

continued

TABLE 2-1 Continued

Surveillance System	Strengths	Limitations	Use During COVID
COVID-19 Vaccine Pregnancy Registry[#]	Active follow-up of pregnancy and infant outcomes Longitudinal monitoring through pregnancy and postpartum periods Ability to link self-reported outcomes with medical records Potentially important system for persons excluded from clinical trials	Potential selection bias (voluntary enrollment) Sensitive data restricting public availability of individual-level data Outcomes dependent on participant retention and data completeness No unvaccinated persons for comparison	Followed thousands of vaccinated pregnant individuals; among first sources of pregnancy outcome data used in ACIP safety decisions

NOTES: * Indicates systems enhanced during the COVID response; # indicates systems newly created specifically for COVID vaccine safety monitoring. AE = adverse event; AESI = adverse event of special interest; CISA = Clinical Immunization Safety Assessment; EHR = electronic health record; RCA = rapid cycle analysis; VAERS = Vaccine Adverse Event Reporting System; VSD = Vaccine Safety Datalink.
SOURCES: CDC, 2024d,g,h,j; Gee, 2024; Gee et al., 2024; HHS, 2024.

TABLE 2-2 Description of Non-CDC COVID Vaccine Safety Data Sources Relevant to ISO

System/Data Source	Description and Relevance to ISO and COVID
FDA BEST	A surveillance system operated by FDA CBER that uses large-scale claims and EHR data. While not led by CDC ISO, BEST conducted parallel analyses of AESIs (e.g., myocarditis, stroke) during the COVID vaccine rollout. ISO and FDA communicated regularly to align on findings and coordinate regulatory communication.
FDA-Mandated Manufacturer Studies	Postauthorization safety studies required by FDA under EUA or licensure agreements. These included prospective studies on pregnancy, myocarditis, and other AESIs. While conducted independently by manufacturers, results were often shared with CDC ISO and informed ACIP safety deliberations.
VA	VA conducted independent observational studies using its comprehensive EHR system. CDC ISO considered VA findings, including mortality and AESI studies, as complementary evidence in evaluating vaccine safety signals. VA data were also discussed during interagency safety coordination meetings.
International Surveillance (e.g., UK MHRA, Israel MOH, EMA)	International regulators provided some of the earliest safety signal data for events such as myocarditis (Israel) and TTS (EU). CDC ISO used these findings to contextualize U.S. data, prioritize surveillance efforts, and prepare clinical guidance and communication materials.
IHS	IHS collaborated with CDC and FDA to monitor American Indian and Alaska Native populations. While this was not an ISO-led platform, IHS data were used to evaluate safety and coverage in populations underrepresented in VSD.
CMS	CMS data were used in joint CDC–FDA evaluations to assess outcomes such as ischemic stroke in older adults. Though ISO does not directly operate CMS surveillance, these data expanded population coverage for AESI evaluation and contributed to cross-agency safety assessments.
NIA/Brown EHR and CMS Data Collaborative	A collaboration supported by the NIH National Institute on Aging and Brown University, linking CMS claims with EHR data from LTC facilities to evaluate COVID vaccine safety in frail, elderly populations. Though it was independent of ISO, findings were shared with CDC and used to assess AESIs (e.g., thrombotic events, mortality) in nursing home residents—a critical population not fully captured in VSD. This represents NIH's involvement in the interagency safety monitoring enterprise.

NOTES: * Indicates systems enhanced during the COVID response; # indicates systems newly created specifically for COVID vaccine safety monitoring. AE = adverse event; AESI = adverse event of special interest; BEST = Biologics Effectiveness and Safety Initiative; CBER = Center for Biologics Evaluation and Research; CDC = Centers for Disease Control and Prevention; CISA = Clinical Immunization Safety Assessment; CMS = Centers for Medicare & Medicaid Services; EHR = electronic health record; EUA = Emergency Use Authorization; FDA = Food and Drug Administration; IHS = Indian Health Service; LTC = long-term care facility; NIH = National Institutes of Health; VA = Department of Veterans Affairs; VAERS = Vaccine Adverse Event Reporting System; VSD = Vaccine Safety Datalink.
SOURCES: Bardenheier et al., 2021; FDA, 2023, 2024a,c; Shimabukuro and Klein, 2023; Wong et al., 2023.

international partners, and vaccine manufacturers—played a critical role in extending the reach of safety monitoring. These systems contributed complementary datasets, populations, and analytic methods. For example, FDA's BEST Initiative conducted large-scale postauthorization evaluations; VA and the Indian Health Service (IHS) provided insights on specific federal health care populations; CMS enabled timely assessment of risks in older adults (FDA, 2023; Shimabukuro and Klein, 2023); and international surveillance systems helped identify early signals, such as myocarditis and TTS. CMS data from long-term care facilities were also incorporated to enhance monitoring among older adults and high-risk populations, illustrating the potential of interagency collaboration. Manufacturer-led postauthorization studies, required under FDA agreements, also generated targeted safety data, particularly in populations excluded from initial trials (FDA, 2024c). Table 2-2 describes these non-CDC systems and their relevance to ISO's safety monitoring efforts during the COVID vaccination program.

Main Safety Findings Across Monitoring Systems

Throughout the COVID vaccination campaign, U.S. safety monitoring systems collectively identified, assessed, and responded to a broad range of AEs following immunization. This surveillance network—comprising VAERS, VSD, CISA, V-safe, and the V-safe Pregnancy Registry—enabled a multifaceted understanding of vaccine safety across diverse populations and conditions. While each system had unique capabilities and limitations, they worked in concert to detect early signals, estimate or validate risks, and inform timely public health guidance.

Many of the events under surveillance were *prespecified outcomes*, determined before vaccine rollout based on historical vaccine safety concerns, COVID disease complications, or findings from clinical trials. These included anaphylaxis, myocarditis, GBS, and thromboembolic events, such as deep vein thrombosis and pulmonary embolism. For each outcome, CDC and FDA required surveillance programs to apply harmonized case definitions—for example, the CDC working definition for myocarditis, ACIP Tier 1–2 criteria for TTS, and Brighton Collaboration standards for anaphylaxis and GBS—to ensure consistency in case ascertainment across VAERS, VSD, V-safe, and CISA (CDC, 2024g, 2025; Korinthenberg and Sejvar, 2020; Marschner et al., 2023; See, 2021; Sejvar et al., 2011). Prespecification helped prioritize investigations, standardize reporting across systems, and reduce analytic bias. Maximizing the utility of these harmonized definitions depends, in part, on compiling results from safety assessments in a centralized, publicly accessible location. Centralized assessment improves transparency, supports integrated interpretation across systems, and enables both researchers and the public to understand emerging safety findings in a more holistic and accessible way.

Across systems, several consistent findings emerged. Anaphylaxis was one of the earliest signals detected—flagged by VAERS within a week of vaccine rollout, which recorded ≈0.00047 percent of participants self-reporting severe allergic reactions (rash, swelling, dyspnea) on Day 0–1 after dose 1, a proportion that closely matched VAERS case counts, and then clinically evaluated in depth by CISA (Shimabukuro, 2021a). Myocarditis and pericarditis were observed predominantly in young men and boys following mRNA vaccines, especially after dose 2; most cases were reported to be mild and to resolve quickly (Marschner et al., 2023). GBS and TTS were linked primarily to the Janssen vaccine, prompting federal guidance changes and ultimately its withdrawal from the U.S. market (Hanson et al., 2022; Rosenblum et al., 2021; See et al., 2021). No increased risk of death, including from non-COVID causes, was found in any system (Oliver et al., 2022). Evaluations of pregnancy and reproductive outcomes and pediatric vaccination and vaccine coadministration consistently reaffirmed the strong safety profile of COVID vaccines (Moro et al., 2021).

VAERS played a pivotal role in rapid signal detection. Reports of anaphylaxis, myocarditis, TTS, and GBS were identified through it, contributing to regulatory responses and ACIP recommendations (Abara et al., 2023; MacNeil et al., 2021; Oster et al., 2022). Despite its limitations as a spontaneous-event reporting system, VAERS provided valuable data for contextualizing risk. For instance, Oster et al. (2022) analyzed VAERS reports of myocarditis following mRNA COVID vaccination using national vaccine administration data as the denominator, calculated reporting rates, and identified risk to be highest after the second dose in adolescent boys and young men, informing timely ACIP risk–benefit assessments (Gargano et al., 2021). Later (mid-2021 to December 2022), VAERS analytic studies found no disproportionate increased risk of tinnitus in any COVID vaccines (Yih et al., 2024). VAERS data provided some reassurance about lack of pregnancy complications (Moro et al., 2024), and all-cause mortality (Xu et al., 2021). VAERS summaries confirmed that the vast majority of reported AEs were nonserious (Ceacareanu and Wintrob, 2021). As described, for COVID vaccines, national administration data—stratified by age, sex, and product—enabled calculating reported rates, a capability not typically available in passive surveillance. However, these rates should be interpreted with caution, as VAERS remains subject to underreporting, differential reporting, and stimulated reporting, and reported rates do not reflect incidence.

VSD enabled active, large-scale, population-based surveillance and comparative risk evaluations across millions of vaccine recipients at 11 integrated health care sites (CDC, 2024c). It provided robust evidence on AE risks stratified by age, sex, pregnancy status, and underlying health conditions. For example, VSD quantified observed rates of myocarditis at ≈137 cases per million second mRNA doses in boys aged 12–15 versus ≈9.3 per million in girls of the same age and GBS at ≈3.1 cases per million Janssen doses—estimates that informed benefit–risk assessments for specific subgroups (Goddard et al., 2022b; Hanson et al., 2022). VSD studies also confirmed no increased risk of miscarriage, preterm birth, or neonatal complications among vaccinated pregnant individuals (Lipkind et al., 2022) and showed no safety concerns when COVID boosters were coadministered with the seasonal influenza vaccine (Kenigsberg et al., 2023a). Mortality analyses revealed lower non-COVID death rates among vaccinated versus unvaccinated members—likely reflecting healthy-vaccinee bias rather than a protective vaccine effect (Xu et al., 2023).

V-safe collected real-time, participant-reported data on common side effects. It played a key role in characterizing mild to moderate reactogenicity, confirming that symptoms like fatigue, fever, and injection-site pain were frequent but brief (CDC, 2024e; Chapin-Bardales et al., 2021). Although it was less suited for assessing rare or serious events, V-safe helped capture signals like menstrual irregularities and provided critical reassurance regarding the overall vaccine tolerability (Wong et al., 2022). Its main analytic limitation was the absence of an unvaccinated comparator group, which made it difficult to determine whether self-reported events occurred above background rates or varied by underlying health status.

CISA contributed detailed clinical insights through expert case reviews and consultations, particularly for complex or high-stakes AEs, like anaphylaxis, myocarditis, and TTS (Williams et al., 2011). Its adjudicated investigations incorporated chart reviews and laboratory diagnostics, adding diagnostic clarity to rare events. However, because CISA focused on referred or severe cases, findings were not generalizable across the broader population (Gee et al., 2024; Williams et al., 2011). Moreover, for certain syndromes—most notably multisystem inflammatory syndrome in adults or children (MIS-A/MIS-C)—CISA's working definitions required laboratory evidence of recent SARS-CoV-2 infection; while this criterion helped distinguish postinfection pathology from coincidental findings, it also meant that vaccine-associated cases without documented infection could be missed (Cortese et al., 2023).

Together, these coordinated vaccine safety monitoring systems were able to comprehensively evaluate the COVID vaccines and provide estimates of risk for various population subgroups. The interplay of rapid signal detection, in-depth clinical review, and longitudinal population-level analysis enabled a comprehensive evaluation of vaccine safety. These analyses were crucial for informing policy and guiding clinical recommendations, although, as noted, challenges occurred in communicating this knowledge to HCPs and the public, undermining the robustness and excellence of the scientific work. Moreover, the majority of publications of these findings included language that risks were "rare," "mostly mild," and "far outweighed by the benefits of protection" against severe COVID. This reassurance was provided even when formal risk–benefit analyses were not included or referenced. Such vaccine promotion may interfere with the perception of independence of ISO vaccine safety monitoring. A cross-system summary of the major COVID-19 vaccine-safety signals, their principal findings, and surveillance periods is provided in Table 2-3.

TIMELINESS AND COMPLETENESS OF SIGNALS

The scale and urgency of the U.S. COVID vaccination campaign required a responsive, transparent, and scientifically rigorous safety infrastructure. VaST was convened by CDC in October 2020 as an ACIP subcommittee to review vaccine safety data in near real time and advise the full ACIP (Lee, 2021; Markowitz et al., 2024). Meeting as often as weekly during the first 18 months of rollout—and then monthly through 2023—VaST examined findings from VAERS, VSD, V-safe, CISA, and external sources, issuing summary memorandums that informed ACIP votes, CDC Health Alerts, and provider advisories (Rosenblum et al., 2022).

To prioritize surveillance, CDC and FDA jointly published a list of AESIs before mass vaccination began; it drew on historical vaccine risks (e.g., anaphylaxis, GBS), COVID disease complications (e.g., MIS-C), and trial signals (e.g., Bell's palsy) (Gee et al., 2021; Lee, 2021; Markowitz et al., 2024). Prespecification improved consistency across systems, yet the framework remained adaptive: when VAERS and V-safe unearthed unexpected patterns—such as menstrual cycle changes or tinnitus—those outcomes were added to monitoring protocols and VaST agendas (Rosenblum et al., 2022). The detailed decision-making logic for adding or retiring signals, however, is documented only in internal VaST working papers and has not been made publicly available.

Safety signal evaluations closely tracked each phase of the rollout—and the timeliness of VaST briefings became a key operating metric. In its first quarter (December 2020–March 2021), VaST met twice per week and delivered slide-deck summaries to ACIP within 24–48 hours; these were posted on the ACIP website the same day as the public meeting, creating near-real-time transparency (CDC, 2024h; Shimabukuro et al., 2021a). Anaphylaxis illustrates the cadence: VaST reviewed the first 21 VAERS cases on December 19, 2020—3 days after the Pfizer-BioNTech launch—and ACIP discussed the findings in an emergency session the next morning (CDC, 2020), CDC's interim clinical guidance and a rapid MMWR followed within 2 weeks (CDC COVID-Response Team et al., 2021; Shimabukuro et al., 2021a).

TABLE 2-3 Cross-System Summary of Major COVID Vaccine Safety Signals, Principal Findings, and Surveillance Periods

Signal/Syndrome	System	Key Finding Reported	Data-Collection Period	Source
Anaphylaxis	VAERS	10 confirmed cases; rate ≈11.1 per million mRNA doses	Dec. 14 2020–Jan. 18 2021	(Shimabukuro, 2021a)
	V-safe	0.00045 percent self-reported "severe allergic reaction" ≤Day 1	Dec. 14 2020–Jan. 13 2021	(Gee et al., 2021)
	CISA	Anti-PEG IgE not detected in 20 evaluated cases	2021–2022	(Zhou et al., 2023)
GBS	VSD	32.4 cases per 100,000 person-years (RR = 20.6 vs. mRNA)	Feb.–Oct. 2021	(Hanson et al., 2022)
	VAERS	Underestimated true rates; however, more frequently reported (9- to 11fold higher) within 21 days after Janssen vaccine than either mRNA vaccine	Dec. 2020–Jan. 2022	(Abara et al., 2023)
Reactogenicity (local/systemic)	V-safe	91–95 percent injection-site pain; 16–46 percent systemic symptoms	Dec. 2020–Feb. 2021	(Hause et al., 2022c)
Mortality	VAERS	9,201 death reports; no mortality signal detected	Dec. 2020–Nov. 2021	(Day et al., 2023)
	VSD	No increase in non-COVID mortality (RR 0.97)	Dec. 2020–Aug. 2021	(Xu et al., 2024)
MIS-C/MIS-A	CISA	Very rare; ≤5 referred cases met criteria	May 2020–Feb. 2022	(Cortese et al., 2023; Yousaf et al., 2022)
Myocarditis/Pericarditis	VSD	Highest in boys 12–17: up to 150 cases per million second doses	Dec. 2020–Aug. 2022	(Goddard et al., 2022a)
	VAERS	Rates high in boys/young men 12–29	Dec. 2020–Aug. 2021	(Oster et al., 2022)

TABLE 2-3 Continued

Signal/Syndrome	System	Key Finding Reported	Data-Collection Period	Source
Pregnancy Outcomes	VAERS	No safety signals for miscarriage or stillbirth	Dec. 2020–Oct. 2021	(Shimabukuro et al., 2021b)
	VSD	Confirmed no increased risk of miscarriage/preterm birth	Dec. 2020–July 2021	(Lipkind et al., 2022)
TTS	VAERS	Reported rate 3.8 cases per million Janssen doses overall; highest in women aged 30–39	Dec. 2020–Aug. 2021	(See et al., 2021)
	CISA	Reviewed neuroimaging and PF4 ELISA results to support clinical evaluation of TTS cases	Dec. 2020–Aug. 2021	(See et al., 2022)
Anxiety-Related Events	VAERS	Spike in syncope; 61 percent female, median age 36	Apr. 21	(Hause et al., 2021)
Booster Coadministration	VSD	No new AESIs with concurrent flu vaccine or COVID booster	Dec. 2020–Jan. 2023	(Katherine Yih et al., 2023; Kenigsberg et al., 2023b)
Daily Activity Impairment	V-safe	Up to ~30% reported daily activity disruption on Day 1, especially after second dose	Dec. 2020–June 2021	(Rosenblum et al., 2022)
Menstrual Changes	V-safe	1 percent reported cycle irregularity	Dec. 2020–Jan. 2022	(Wong et al., 2022)
Overall Safety	VSD	Generally favorable; no new serious AESIs detected	Dec. 2020–Oct. 2021	(Yih et al., 2023)

NOTE: AESI = adverse event of special interest; CISA = Clinical Immunization Safety Assessment; ELISA = enzyme-linked immunosorbent assay; GBS = Guillain-Barré syndrome; MISC-A/C = multisystem inflammatory syndrome in adults/children; RR= Reporting Rate; TTS = thrombosis with thrombocytopenia syndrome; VAERS = Vaccine Adverse Event Reporting System; VSD = Vaccine Safety Datalink.
SOURCES: Abara et al., 2023; Cortese et al., 2023; Day et al., 2023; Frontera et al., 2022; Gee et al., 2021; Goddard et al., 2022a; Hanson et al., 2022; Hause et al., 2021, 2022c; Kenigsberg et al., 2023b; Lipkind et al., 2022; Oster et al., 2022; Rosenblum et al., 2022; See et al., 2021, 2022; Shimabukuro, 2021a,b; Wong et al., 2022; Xu et al., 2024; Yih et al., 2023; Yousaf et al., 2022; Zhou et al., 2023.

Early all-cause-mortality data were brought to VaST on January 27, 2021; although VAERS counts suggested no excess deaths, the group immediately commissioned RCAs in VSD and previewed interim results to ACIP on March 1, 2021 (ACIP, 2021b, 2021c). Peer-reviewed VSD papers released in 2021, 2022, and 2024 all corroborated the absence of a vaccine-associated mortality signal (Klein et al., 2021; Xu et al., 2023, 2024).

Overall, VaST's ability to convene within days, circulate presentations in under 48 hours, and present data important for ACIP decision making—often within hours or days—proved critical for rapid, evidence-based updates to CDC guidance and provider alerts (ACIP, 2021d).

Pregnancy safety was an early and high-priority focus of COVID vaccine monitoring efforts, including through a registry that operated during the early rollout but was discontinued in 2023 (Gee et al., 2024; Madni et al., 2024). Ongoing monitoring of pregnancy outcomes continues through systems such as VSD and VAERS. With clinical trials excluding pregnant individuals, CDC launched the V-safe COVID-19 Vaccine Pregnancy Registry in December 2020 (CDC, 2024f). VaST convened a pregnancy-focused session in February 2021 that reviewed the first reports from V-safe and VAERS (Lee and Hopkins, 2021). Subsequent evaluations across V-safe, VAERS, and VSD consistently found no increased risk of miscarriage, preterm birth, stillbirth, or neonatal complications among the vaccinated (Lipkind et al., 2022; Shimabukuro et al., 2021b; Zauche et al., 2021). In parallel, menstrual changes—though not prespecified—were examined after public concern: VaST reviewed V-safe data showing ~1 percent of female participants reporting menstrual irregularities, and VSD analyses found postmenopausal bleeding to be uncommon (Wong et al., 2022).

For newer or rarer safety signals, timeliness depended on how quickly robust data could be gathered and analyzed. TTS linked to the Janssen vaccine was first identified internally by CDC and FDA on April 9, 2021, reviewed by VaST on April 12, less than 2 months after the EUA, and triggered a nationwide "pause" announced on April 13, 2021, followed by an emergency ACIP meeting on April 14 and updated vaccine recommendations issued on April 23 (FDA, 2021; MacNeil et al., 2021; See et al., 2021; Shay et al., 2021).

Myocarditis associated with mRNA vaccines in young men and boys surfaced in VAERS and VSD in May 2021. VAERS reported rates were close to background, suggesting a possible problem, given that reporting to VAERS is generally incomplete. Accumulating U.S. and international data—along with CISA cardiology consultations—led CDC to issue interim clinical guidance on May 17, 2021 and ACIP to hold a dedicated review on June 23, 2021 (CDC, 2025a; MacNeil et al., 2021; Shimabukuro, 2022).

GBS following Janssen vaccination was first discussed by VaST on June 10, 2021. Elevated VAERS reporting rates were later confirmed in a

VSD RCA released to ACIP on December 16, 2021, and published in 2022, underpinning ACIP's January 5, 2022, recommendation to preferentially use mRNA vaccines (Alimchandani, 2021; Hanson et al., 2022).

Evaluations of coadministration with influenza vaccines began in autumn 2021; VaST and VSD reviews found no serious safety concerns, although mild increases in systemic reactogenicity were noted (Hause et al., 2022c; Kenigsberg et al., 2023b).

As vaccines expanded to children and boosters, new formulations and recommendations were accompanied by ongoing VaST review. Between November 2020 and April 2023, VaST held regular meetings and presented 22 safety assessments to ACIP, supporting benefit–risk evaluations and informing vaccine policy. In April 2023, its responsibilities transitioned back to the ACIP COVID-19 Vaccines Work Group as part of a return to routine safety assessment procedures.

Bivalent mRNA boosters, introduced in August 2022, were evaluated in a joint VAERS and V-safe analysis of >22 million administered doses that revealed no new safety concerns (Hause et al., 2022b).

In January 2023, VSD detected a transient statistical signal for ischemic stroke in adults ≥65 years after the Pfizer bivalent booster, but it disappeared in updated VSD runs and was not corroborated by VAERS, CMS, or international data (FDA, 2023; Shimabukuro and Klein, 2023).

Additional topics reviewed included pediatric safety after primary and booster doses in children 6 months and older (no new signals) (CDC, 2024i; Hause et al., 2023), tinnitus (no association confirmed in VSD) (Yih et al., 2024), and concurrent COVID/flu vaccination (no serious AESIs, minor uptick in reactogenicity) (Kenigsberg et al., 2023a). Throughout its operation, VaST reviewed data from a range of sources, including VAERS, VSD, V-safe, the pregnancy registry, and other monitoring systems external to CDC, such as Biologics Effectiveness and Safety (BEST), VA, DoD, and IHS. CISA contributed technical consultation and clinical insights.

Although peer-reviewed manuscripts sometimes appeared months later, key safety findings were typically communicated first through MMWR bulletins, ACIP slide decks, and clinician listserv alerts, ensuring that frontline providers and the public received timely guidance while full-scale studies were still underway.

Finally, the timelines for generating and disseminating results varied by system and outcome severity. Preliminary analyses for high-priority signals were typically presented to ACIP within days or weeks—anaphylaxis on December 12, 2020 (ACIP, 2020), TTS on April 23, 2021 (Shimabukuro, 2021b), myocarditis on June 23, 2021 (ACIP, 2021d), and the ischemic-stroke assessment for Pfizer's bivalent booster on January 26, 2023 (Shimabukuro, 2023a)—well before any peer-reviewed papers appeared. VSD publications on acute outcomes, like myocarditis, typically followed within

6–12 months; more complex evaluations—especially of pregnancy or long-term effects—required 1.5–2.5 years. VAERS descriptive studies appeared sooner, providing early context and reassurance, while CISA's in-depth clinical investigations, though slower to publish, still informed rapid decision making through real-time expert consultation.

These processes underscore the importance of both structure and flexibility in national vaccine safety evaluation. Prespecified outcomes provided a foundation for proactive monitoring, while system adaptability allowed for investigating unanticipated concerns—ensuring that safety questions were addressed promptly and transparently during an evolving public health crisis.

OPPORTUNITY/ATTENTION COSTS

The ISO research agenda necessitates deliberate tradeoffs in resource allocation—both at the systems level and in the prioritization of specific safety signal investigations. Effective navigation of these tradeoffs, particularly in dynamic public health contexts, such as the COVID vaccine safety investigations, requires procedural readiness and access to integrated information that can support accelerated decision making and translating this knowledge for the population.

At the systems level, ISO's rapid incorporation of long-term care data (CDC, 2025b) to augment existing surveillance platforms illustrated the benefits of interagency collaboration in generating timely and novel insights—an uncommon but highly effective example of cross-agency coordination. At the level of individual safety signals, the timeliness of VaST report generation, as summarized in Table 2-3, demonstrates responsiveness when signals are actively pursued. However, the absence of communication regarding decisions to defer or decline investigations of certain potential signals (e.g., menstrual irregularities) may have diminished public trust, leaving a vacuum filled by speculation and unmoderated discourse.

Limitations and Opportunities for a Unified Vaccine Safety Infrastructure

The committee was not provided information on ISO's internal decision-making processes for determining which safety analyses to pursue, nor was it given access to data on how its budget was allocated. Please see Chapter 1 for details. Despite these limitations, internal reviews and independent evaluations have examined ISO's surveillance architecture, including its operational advantages and inherent constraints.

Although certain avenues for accessing vaccination status data were expanded during the PHE—for example, through temporary agreements with CMS and national pharmacy chains—the absence of a comprehensive, federally mandated vaccination reporting policy remains a significant obstacle to integrated safety surveillance (U.S. GAO, 2021). Each state, territory, and local jurisdiction governs its own Immunization Information System (IIS), and these vary widely in technical functionality, legal authority, and scope of reporting requirements (CDC, 2024j). While IISs are primarily used for tracking vaccine administration, their data can enhance safety monitoring by providing accurate denominator data for reported rates and supporting linkage to AE reports across systems. Although most jurisdictions responded to CDC's COVID data-sharing requests—enabled in part by federal control of vaccine supply under EUA—many lacked bidirectional interoperability with hospitals, pharmacies, long-term care facilities, and nontraditional vaccination sites, such as mass clinics and community pop-ups. These settings were central to reaching uninsured and underserved populations yet often fell outside routine health data streams and did not consistently transmit records into IISs or systems like VSD. In some states, data from these sources were submitted via spreadsheets and uploaded manually, leading to time lags, reduced data quality, and missed opportunities to link to safety outcomes.

Although CDC has issued functional standards for core IIS data elements—including patient demographics, lot number, and provider details—implementation is voluntary and varies by jurisdiction (CDC, 2024k). The EUA for COVID vaccines temporarily required providers to report administered doses and AEs to federal authorities (CDC, 2024f), which allowed systems like VAERS to calculate reported rates of adverse events of special interest (AESIs) with greater accuracy. However, these mandates did not extend to other vaccines or persist beyond the PHE. Without a national immunization registry or harmonized legal and technical infrastructure, the United States remains limited in its ability to integrate vaccination records—particularly from uninsured or nontraditional care settings—into a comprehensive safety surveillance framework. Structural challenges—most notably the lack of a coordinated, department-wide strategy and infrastructure for generating and integrating vaccine safety and effectiveness data—continue to limit the efficiency, impact, and scalability of CDC and HHS investments (Bauchau et al., 2023).

Stakeholders, including those providing public input during ACIP meetings (e.g., April 2021, Scott Razen, CUNY), have highlighted the opportunity for transitioning from a patchwork of systems toward a modern, integrated, active, and nationally representative surveillance system (ACIP, 2021a; Razen, 2021). ISO has demonstrated capacity for leveraging partnerships with platforms funded by the National Institutes of Health, CMS, and private-sector entities (e.g., pharmacies) to access data not traditionally available within VSD (Bauchau et al., 2023; Haendel et al., 2021). This underscores the potential for coinvestment in a unified postauthorization/postmarketing system capable of evaluating both safety and effectiveness of vaccines, devices, and therapeutics. Opportunities for optimization include integrating benefit–risk assessments within a single infrastructure, deduplicating parallel data streams and redundant procurements, and creating a "data sandbox" of deidentified assets to support cross-agency analytics.

Transparent Coordination Across CDC and Non-CDC Systems

Enhanced transparency in the governance of surveillance systems and safety signal workflows is essential. This includes increased public input—particularly from communities with specific concerns—and clear communication regarding system and signal prioritization criteria. Rather than consolidating into a single data source, a modernized approach should preserve multiple, independent input streams while integrating findings and communications into a unified, transparent, and accessible framework. For example, complementary analyses from the passive VAERS and active VSD during the investigation of myocarditis following mRNA vaccination offered both rapid signal detection and structured follow-up analysis, illustrating the value of diverse inputs with coordinated interpretation (Goddard et al., 2022b; Marschner et al., 2023; Shimabukuro, 2022). Ensuring high standards of evidence quality across systems—and synthesizing findings in a coordinated voice for vaccine risk assessment—will strengthen both public trust and scientific rigor in safety assessments.

While pandemic-era adaptations showcased CDC ISO's ability to leverage partnerships with FDA, CMS, academic centers, and private-sector entities, the absence of a durable, high-level oversight body limited the strategic coordination of safety efforts across federal and state platforms. Improved alignment, via interagency agreements, shared technical standards, and joint prioritization of safety signal evaluation will be essential to optimize resource use, eliminate redundancies, and improve analytic transparency in future PHEs.

The Global Vaccine Data Network (GVDN) played a significant complementary role in the global evaluation of COVID vaccine safety. Despite a slow start due to early funding limitations, GVDN implemented standardized protocols to conduct RCAs and background rate estimation studies across an international network that included New Zealand, Indonesia, Argentina, the African COVID-19 Vaccine Safety Surveillance system (South Africa, Mali, Ghana, Nigeria, Ethiopia, Kenya, Malawi, and Mozambique), Australia (Victoria and New South Wales), Canada (British Columbia and Ontario), Denmark, Finland, the Republic of Korea, Hong Kong, and multiple Vaccine Monitoring Collaboration for Europe sites, including the

United Kingdom and Spain (Valencia and Catalonia). Published studies from the network have provided foundational estimates of background rates for AESIs (Phillips et al., 2023), multinational risk estimates for GBS (Nasreen et al., 2025), and large-scale cohort analyses involving nearly 100 million individuals (Faksova et al., 2024). A signal for acute disseminated encephalomyelitis identified in this cohort was validated in a follow-up study (Morgan et al., 2024). Additional GVDN studies of TTS and myocarditis/pericarditis are forthcoming. While these efforts involved U.S.-based collaborators and contributed important scientific insights, this report focuses on systems primarily developed and operated by CDC, HHS, or directly funded federal partners. Nonetheless, GVDN offers a compelling model for international collaboration, harmonized protocols, and large-scale signal detection.

Technology Investment and Ecosystem Coordination

Optimizing the informational value derived from the surveillance ecosystem will require sustained investments in technological infrastructure and intersystem coordination. Operational costs for individual systems are not disclosed, and clarity is insufficient regarding population-level overlap across CDC's active-surveillance platforms and those of partner agencies. This lack of transparency impedes efforts to assess resource efficiency, identify gaps in demographic or geographic coverage, and reduce redundancy. Improved interoperability and shared technical standards across platforms—such as those operated by CDC, CMS, FDA, and others—could enhance scalability, accelerate analytic turnaround, and support coordinated responses during future PHEs (CDC, 2024l).

The PHE demonstrated what is possible when legal and technical barriers to data access are lifted. Under the PREP Act and EUAs (see Chapter 1), CDC and its partners were able to access vaccination data from pharmacy chains, long-term care providers, and health insurers; link immunization records with AE data across systems; and generate timely, high-resolution safety signals (CDC, 2024c; FDA, 2024b). These flexibilities enabled calculating reported AE rates with denominators, even for populations often excluded from traditional health system surveillance.

Now that these authorities have expired (Hickey, 2025), many structural constraints have returned. No federal mandate exists for real-time vaccination data reporting outside of emergencies, and state-level IISs remain highly variable in legal authority, technical standards, and bidirectional connectivity. Fragmented governance, inconsistent adoption of interoperability frameworks, and limited mechanisms for accessing data from uninsured individuals or nontraditional vaccination sites reduce the completeness and utility of national safety surveillance. Without sustained legal and technical infrastructure, the country remains underprepared to replicate this level of surveillance performance outside a declared emergency.

To ensure sustained preparedness, a dedicated cross-agency governance structure is needed to coordinate vaccine safety monitoring activities across CDC, FDA, CMS, NIH, and state public health systems. Such coordination should preserve system independence while enabling shared analytic priorities, streamlined signal evaluation protocols, and unified communication of findings.

Signal Investigation Prioritization

Investment decisions must also address the intensity with which specific safety signals are investigated and updated. While the initial lists are typically grounded in prior evidence and included in surveillance protocols, the criteria and processes by which new signals are nominated, prioritized, or deprioritized remain opaque. In interviews, most CISA researchers described priority-setting as a "black box," noting limited involvement and advocating for earlier and more transparent collaboration with CDC in shaping research agendas. One researcher called to develop structured mechanisms to incorporate academic expertise and methodological innovation within a coordinated federal framework, rather than relying solely on traditional CDC-led processes (Westat, 2025; Appendix C).

System-specific limitations further constrain signal investigation. For instance, vaccine safety experts reported that VAERS lacked the infrastructure for systematic AE follow-up, and that the initial design of V-safe—intended to support direct response to all reports—was quickly overwhelmed, limiting its utility for sustained monitoring. These constraints diminish the capacity of surveillance systems to support iterative investigation of safety signals. Ensuring the ability to respond to emerging post-authorization data will require strengthened mechanisms to identify and escalate signals meriting longitudinal, methodologically rigorous follow-up beyond the inherent constraints of passive surveillance systems and even VSD's limited subpopulation stratification (Westat, 2025; Appendix C).

ADDITIONAL UNPUBLISHED, REAL-TIME FINDINGS/SAFETY ASSESSMENTS

VaST and ACIP Presentations

Throughout the COVID vaccine rollout, ACIP—a federal advisory body responsible for developing immunization recommendations—served as the primary venue for public presentation and deliberation of vaccine safety data. CDC established VaST in November 2020 as a rapid-review body composed of independent safety experts. VaST met regularly—sometimes weekly—to assess preliminary data from multiple surveillance platforms, including VAERS, VSD, and V-safe, and inputs from the CISA network and external sources, such as international partners. Its assessments were used to inform ACIP discussions about benefit–risk balance, especially during time-sensitive decisions related to EUA expansion, booster eligibility, and pediatric vaccination (Gee et al., 2021; Shimabukuro et al., 2021a).

ISO played a foundational role in enabling these assessments. It is responsible for managing and coordinating the federal postauthorization vaccine safety monitoring infrastructure, including data collection, curation, and preliminary analysis across surveillance systems. While ISO does not make recommendations or conduct formal benefit–risk assessments, it supports ACIP and VaST by providing timely, high-quality safety data and technical interpretation. These data are integrated into ACIP's structured Evidence to Recommendation framework, which weighs safety alongside other domains, such as disease burden, vaccine efficacy, acceptability, and equity. The distinct yet complementary roles of ISO (data generation) and ACIP (policy recommendation) supported efforts to make decisions more transparent, evidence based, and appropriately contextualized.

In addition to prespecified AESIs, VaST and ACIP rapidly reviewed real-time safety signals arising during the vaccination campaign. These included both known concerns—like myocarditis and anaphylaxis—and emerging issues, such as tinnitus and coadministration with influenza vaccines. Table 2-4 summarizes selected signals, highlighting the timelines from first internal review, to public communication (e.g., ACIP meetings or FDA warnings), to peer-reviewed publication; ACIP meetings often provided the earliest public transparency on safety signals—sometimes months ahead of formal studies—reinforcing the importance of this advisory process as a mechanism for real-time communication of vaccine safety data.

CONCLUSION

The COVID PHE placed extraordinary demands on ISO, requiring rapid data collection, evaluation, and communication of emerging vaccine safety signals. The integrated infrastructure deployed—spanning passive systems, like VAERS, active platforms, like VSD and V-safe, expert consultation from CISA, and specialized initiatives, such as the COVID-19 Pregnancy Registry—enabled a scale and depth of vaccine safety surveillance without precedent in U.S. public health enterprises. Taken together, these systems supported real-time risk assessment, informed regulatory and clinical recommendations, and guided programmatic decisions.

However, the pandemic exposed structural challenges that, if addressed, could position ISO to be even more effective in future public health responses. As stated in Chapter 1, the committee is applying guiding principles to its

TABLE 2-4 Selected COVID Vaccine Safety Signals—Timeline from Initial VaST Review to Public Disclosure, Peer-Reviewed Evidence, and Action

Safety Signal	VaST First Internal Review	First Public Communication	First Peer-Reviewed Paper	Outcome
Anaphylaxis (mRNA vaccines)	12/19/2020	ACIP emergency session (20 Dec. 2020, open webcast)	CDC RESPONSE *MMWR* 70:46 (Jan. 15, 2021)	~11 cases/million doses; reinforced screening & 15-min observation, no product pause
TTS (Ad26.COV2.S)	4/9/2021	CDC/FDA joint "pause" media statement (Apr. 13, 2021)	MacNeil et al. (2021)	3–4 cases/million (mainly women < 50 y); 10-day pause, warning added to EUA
Myocarditis/ pericarditis (mRNA)	5/24/2021	ACIP public meeting (23 Jun 2021) slides "Update on COVID-19-vaccine safety"	Gargano et al. (2021)	Highest in male recipients 12–29 y (≈70/ million second doses); clinical guidance & product fact-sheet update
GBS (Ad26.COV2.S)	6/10/2021	FDA Fact-sheet revision & press release (Jul. 12, 2021)	Woo et al. (2021)	Excess ≈ 17 cases/million; ACIP (Dec. 2021) prefers mRNA products
Pregnancy outcomes	2/1/2021	ACIP safety update on pregnancy registry (01 Mar 2021) minutes	Shimabukuro et al. (2021b)	Miscarriage, stillbirth, neonatal outcomes within expected background—reassurance, formal recommendation issued
Simultaneous COVID booster + flu shot	10/14/2021	ACIP discussion on coadministration (Oct. 20, 2021)	Hause et al. (2022c)	Mild ↑ systemic reactogenicity; no serious AESI—concurrent vaccination allowed
Tinnitus	11/14/2022	ACIP VaST briefing (slides posted same day)	Yih et al. (2024)	No disproportional reporting or VSD signal; no label change, monitoring continues

NOTE: ACIP = Advisory Committee on Immunization Practices; CDC = Centers for Disease Control and Prevention; CISA = Clinical Immunization Safety Assessment; EUA = Emergency Use Authorization; FDA = Food and Drug Administration; GBS = Guillain-Barré syndrome; MMWR = *Morbidity and Mortality Weekly Report*; TTS = thrombosis with thrombocytopenia syndrome; VA = Department of Veterans Affairs; VAERS = Vaccine Adverse Event Reporting System; VaST = Vaccines Safety Technical (work group); VSD = Vaccine Safety Datalink.
SOURCES: CDC COVID-Response Team et al., 2021; Gargano et al., 2021; Hause et al., 2022c; MacNeil et al., 2021; Shimabukuro et al., 2021b; Woo et al., 2021; Yih et al., 2024.

assessment and recommendations. Its conclusion of ISO's data monitoring and assessment activities is organized following those principles.

Relevance: ISO's monitoring activities were often shaped by urgent public health priorities, but the absence of a clearly articulated mission or long-term strategic plan limited external visibility into how those were determined or adjusted. Ensuring the relevance of ISO's work will depend on formal mechanisms to incorporate input from health professionals, public health stakeholders, and the broader public into planning, prioritization, and communication strategies.

Credibility: The scientific credibility and excellence of ISO's surveillance outputs was supported by consistent use of robust epidemiological methods and transparent engagement in public forums, such as ACIP meetings. However, variation in risk estimates across platforms and the lack of a centralized, accessible portfolio of risk information, tailored to technical and lay audiences, made it difficult for many to interpret the data consistently. More standardized communication tools—such as plain-language summaries, clearly labeled system-specific findings, and consistent risk metrics—could improve clarity and usability. Additionally, where possible, ISO should adopt standardized risk-reporting formats that incorporate relevant subgroup analyses to facilitate clearer public understanding and comparison of findings.

Improvement and Innovation: The rapid deployment of new tools during the PHE also underscores ISO's capacity for continuous improvement and innovation. Developing structured processes to evaluate and integrate emerging scientific methods, data technologies, and communication research could support more agile and forward-looking safety surveillance. Sustaining these efforts beyond emergency response will require dedicated resources, coordination across federal systems, and the flexibility to evolve alongside novel vaccine platforms.

Independence: Finally, the integrity of ISO's work depends on its ability to operate with independence—producing data and evaluations that are scientifically rigorous and insulated from policy or promotional influence. While ISO collaborates across CDC and HHS to inform immunization efforts, independence requires that its analyses and communications remain clearly distinct from vaccine advocacy and policymaking. Ensuring this separation—articulated in ISO's mission, decision-making, functions and communications—will be essential to maintain clarity of purpose and protect the scientific objectivity of ISO's work.

The COVID pandemic reinforced the indispensable role of ISO's surveillance systems in identifying, evaluating, and communicating vaccine risks. As future challenges emerge, strengthening ISO's capacity through transparent planning, inclusive stakeholder engagement, methodological rigor, and clear independence will be essential for advancing a robust, coordinated vaccine safety infrastructure.

REFERENCES

Abara, W. E., J. Gee, P. Marquez, J. Woo, T. R. Myers, A. DeSantis, J. A. G. Baumblatt, E. J. Woo, D. Thompson, N. Nair, J. R. Su, T. T. Shimabukuro, and D. K. Shay. 2023. Reports of Guillain-Barre Syndrome after COVID-19 vaccination in the United States. *JAMA Netw Open* 6(2):e2253845.

ACIP (Advisory Committee on Immunization Practices). 2020. Meeting of the Advisory Committee on Immunization Practices (ACIP), December 11–12, 2020, summary minutes.

ACIP. 2021a. *Advisory Committee on Immunization Practices (ACIP) summary report: April 23, 2021.* Atlanta, GA.

ACIP. 2021b. *Meeting of the Advisory Committee on Immunization Practices (ACIP) February 28–March 1, 2021 summary report.* Atlanta, GA.

ACIP. 2021c. *Meeting of the Advisory Committee on Immunization Practices (ACIP), January 27, 2021: Summary minutes.* Atlanta, GA.

ACIP. 2021d. *Meeting of the Advisory Committee on Immunization Practices (ACIP), June 23, 2021 summary minutes.* Atlanta, GA.

Alimchandani, M. 2021. Guillain-Barré Syndrome (GBS) after Janssen COVID-19 vaccine: Vaccine Adverse Event Reporting System (VAERS), Atlanta, GA.

Anderson, S. 2020. CBER plans for monitoring COVID-19 vaccine safety and effectiveness. Paper read at Vaccines and Related Biological Products Advisory Committee (VRBPAC) meeting, October 22, 2020, Silver Spring, MD.

Baden, L. R., H. M. El Sahly, B. Essink, K. Kotloff, S. Frey, R. Novak, D. Diemert, S. A. Spector, N. Rouphael, C. B. Creech, J. McGettigan, S. Khetan, N. Segall, J. Solis, A. Brosz, C. Fierro, H. Schwartz, K. Neuzil, L. Corey, P. Gilbert, H. Janes, D. Follmann, M. Marovich, J. Mascola, L. Polakowski, J. Ledgerwood, B. S. Graham, H. Bennett, R. Pajon, C. Knightly, B. Leav, W. Deng, H. Zhou, S. Han, M. Ivarsson, J. Miller, T. Zaks, and C. S. Group. 2021. Efficacy and safety of the mRNA-1273 SARS-CoV-2 vaccine. *N Engl J Med* 384(5):403–416.

Bardenheier, B. H., S. Gravenstein, C. Blackman, R. Gutman, I. N. Sarkar, R. A. Feifer, E. M. White, K. McConeghy, A. Nanda, and V. Mor. 2021. Adverse events following mRNA SARS-CoV-2 vaccination among US nursing home residents. *Vaccine* 39(29):3844-3851.

Bauchau, V., K. Davis, S. Frise, C. Jouquelet-Royer, and J. Wilkins. 2023. Real-world monitoring of COVID-19 vaccines: An industry expert view on the successes, challenges, and future opportunities. *Drug Saf* 46(4):327–333.

Black, S., J. Eskola, C. A. Siegrist, N. Halsey, N. MacDonald, B. Law, E. Miller, N. Andrews, J. Stowe, D. Salmon, K. Vannice, H. S. Izurieta, A. Akhtar, M. Gold, G. Oselka, P. Zuber, D. Pfeifer, and C. Vellozzi. 2009. Importance of background rates of disease in assessment of vaccine safety during mass immunisation with pandemic H1N1 influenza vaccines. *Lancet* 374(9707):2115–2122.

CDC (Centers for Disease Control and Prevention). 2020. ACIP meeting slides: December 19–20, 2020. https://archive.cdc.gov/www_cdc_gov/vaccines/acip/meetings/slides-2020-12-19-20.html (accessed August 7, 2025).

CDC. 2021. ACIP COVID-19 vaccine safety technical (VAST) work group: May 17, 2021, VAST assessment of thrombosis with thrombocytopenia syndrome (TTS) after Johnson & Johnson's Janssen COVID-19 vaccine. https://archive.cdc.gov/www_cdc_gov/vaccines/acip/work-groups-vast/report-2021-05-17.html (accessed August 7, 2025).

CDC. 2023. *COVID-19 vaccination reporting for healthcare personnel: NHSN module operational guidance.* Centers for Disease Control and Prevention.

CDC. 2024a. Vaccine Adverse Event Reporting System (VAERS). https://wonder.cdc.gov/wonder/help/vaers.html (accessed August 7, 2025).

CDC. 2024b. COVID-19 vaccination program provider requirements and support. https://www.cdc.gov/vaccines/covid-19/vaccination-provider-support.html (accessed August 7, 2025).

CDC. 2024c. Vaccine Safety Datalink (VSD). https://www.cdc.gov/vaccine-safety-systems/vsd/ (accessed August, 7, 2025).

CDC. 2024d. Clinical immunization safety assessment (CISA) project. https://www.cdc.gov/vaccine-safety-systems/hcp/cisa/index.html (accessed August 7, 2025).

CDC. 2024e. About V-safe. https://www.cdc.gov/vaccine-safety-systems/v-safe/index.html (accessed September 10, 2025).

CDC. 2024f. V-safe COVID-19 vaccine pregnancy registry. https://www.cdc.gov/vaccine-safety-systems/monitoring/covid-preg-reg.html (accessed August 7, 2025).

CDC. 2024g. Myocarditis and pericarditis after mRNA COVID-19 vaccination. https://www.cdc.gov/vaccines/covid-19/clinical-considerations/myocarditis.html (accessed August 7, 2025).

CDC. 2024h. Advisory Committee on Immunization Practices (ACIP) meeting agendas. https://www.cdc.gov/acip/meetings/agendas.html (accessed August 7, 2025).

CDC. 2024i. Evidence to recommendation framework (EtR) for use of COVID-19 vaccines in the 2024–2025 formula for persons 6 months of age and older. https://www.cdc.gov/acip/evidence-to-recommendations/covid-19-2024-2025-6-months-and-older-etr.html (accessed August 7, 2025).

CDC. 2024j. Immunization information systems (IIS): Policy and legislation. https://www.cdc.gov/iis/policy-legislation/index.html (accessed August 7, 2025).

CDC. 2024k. Immunization information systems (IIS): Core data elements. https://www.cdc.gov/iis/core-data-elements/index.html (accessed August 7, 2025).

CDC. 2024l. CDC data modernization efforts accelerate nation's ability to detect and rapidly respond to health threats. https://www.cdc.gov/media/releases/2024/p0411-CDC-data-modernization.html (accessed August 7, 2025).

CDC. 2025a. *Interim clinical considerations for use of COVID-19 vaccines in the United States.* Centers for Disease Control and Prevention.

CDC. 2025b. *Long-term care facilities (LTCF) component.* https://www.cdc.gov/nhsn/ltc/index.html (accessed August 8, 2025).

CDC and FDA (CDC COVID Response Team and Food and Drug Administration). 2021. Allergic reactions including anaphylaxis after receipt of the first dose of Pfizer-BioNTech COVID-19 vaccine—United States, December 14–23, 2020. *MMWR Morb Mortal Wkly Rep* 70(2):46–51.

Ceacareanu, A. C., and Z. A. P. Wintrob. 2021. Summary of COVID-19 vaccine-related reports in the vaccine adverse event reporting system. *J Res Pharm Pract* 10(3):107–113.

Chapin-Bardales, J., T. Myers, J. Gee, D. K. Shay, P. Marquez, J. Baggs, B. Zhang, C. Licata, and T. T. Shimabukuro. 2021. Reactogenicity within 2 weeks after mRNA COVID-19 vaccines: Findings from the CDC V-safe surveillance system. *Vaccine* 39(48):7066–7073.

Chen, R. T., J. W. Glasser, P. H. Rhodes, R. L. Davis, W. E. Barlow, R. S. Thompson, J. P. Mullooly, S. B. Black, H. R. Shinefield, C. M. Vadheim, S. M. Marcy, J. I. Ward, R. P. Wise, S. G. Wassilak, and S. C. Hadler. 1997. Vaccine safety datalink project: A new tool for improving vaccine safety monitoring in the United States. The Vaccine Safety Datalink Team. *Pediatrics* 99(6):765–773.

Cortese, M. M., A. W. Taylor, L. J. Akinbami, A. Thames-Allen, A. R. Yousaf, A. P. Campbell, S. A. Maloney, T. A. Harrington, E. G. Anyalechi, D. Munshi, S. Kamidani, C. R. Curtis, D. W. McCormick, M. A. Staat, K. M. Edwards, C. B. Creech, O. Museru, P. Marquez, D. Thompson, J. R. Su, E. P. Schlaudecker, and K. R. Broder. 2023. Surveillance for multisystem inflammatory syndrome in US children aged 5-11 years who received Pfizer-BioNTech COVID-19 vaccine, November 2021 through March 2022. *J Infect Dis* 228(2):143–148.

Das, M. K. 2023. Adverse events following immunization: The known unknowns and black box: Based on 10th Dr. I. C. Verma Excellence Award for Young Pediatricians delivered as oration on 9th Oct. 2022. *Indian J Pediatr* 90(8):817–825.

Davis, R. L. 2013. Vaccine safety surveillance systems: Critical elements and lessons learned in the development of the US vaccine safety datalink's rapid cycle analysis capabilities. *Pharmaceutics* 5(1):168–178.

Day, B., D. Menschik, D. Thompson, C. Jankosky, J. Su, P. Moro, C. Zinderman, K. Welsh, R. B. Dimova, and N. Nair. 2023. Reporting rates for VAERS death reports following COVID-19 vaccination, December 14, 2020–November 17, 2021. *Pharmacoepidemiol Drug Saf* 32(7):763–772.

Faksova, K., D. Walsh, Y. Jiang, J. Griffin, A. Phillips, A. Gentile, J. C. Kwong, K. Macartney, M. Naus, Z. Grange, S. Escolano, G. Sepulveda, A. Shetty, A. Pillsbury, C. Sullivan, Z. Naveed, N. Z. Janjua, N. Giglio, J. Perala, S. Nasreen, H. Gidding, P. Hovi, T. Vo, F. Cui, L. Deng, L. Cullen, M. Artama, H. Lu, H. J. Clothier, K. Batty, J. Paynter, H. Petousis-Harris, J. Buttery, S. Black, and A. Hviid. 2024. COVID-19 vaccines and adverse events of special interest: A multinational Global Vaccine Data Network (GVDN) cohort study of 99 million vaccinated individuals. *Vaccine* 42(9):2200–2211.

FDA (Food and Drug Administration). 2017. *Final assessment of the FDA sentinel initiative.* Food and Drug Administration.

FDA. 2021. FDA and CDC lift recommended pause on Johnson & Johnson (Janssen) COVID-19 vaccine use following thorough safety review. https://www.fda.gov/news-events/press-announcements/fda-and-cdc-lift-recommended-pause-johnson-johnson-janssen-covid-19-vaccine-use-following-thorough (accessed August 7, 2025).

FDA. 2023. CDC and FDA identify a preliminary COVID-19 vaccine safety signal for persons aged 65 years and older. https://www.fda.gov/vaccines-blood-biologics/safety-availability-biologics/cdc-and-fda-identify-preliminary-covid-19-vaccine-safety-signal-persons-aged-65-years-and-older (accessed September 3, 2025).

FDA. 2024a. CBER biologics effectiveness and safety (BEST) system. https://www.fda.gov/vaccines-blood-biologics/safety-availability-biologics/cber-biologics-effectiveness-and-safety-best-system (accessed August 7, 2025).

FDA. 2024b. Emergency use authorization. https://www.fda.gov/emergency-preparedness-and-response/mcm-legal-regulatory-and-policy-framework/emergency-use-authorization (accessed August 7, 2025).

FDA. 2024c. Postmarketing requirements and commitments: Introduction. https://www.fda.gov/drugs/guidance-compliance-regulatory-information/postmarketing-requirements-and-commitments-introduction (accessed August 7, 2025).

Frontera, J. A., A. A. Tamborska, M. F. Doheim, D. Garcia-Azorin, H. Gezegen, A. Guekht, A. H. K. Yusof Khan, M. Santacatterina, J. Sejvar, K. T. Thakur, E. Westenberg, A. S. Winkler, E. Beghi, and Contributors from the Global COVID-19 Neuro Research Coalition. 2022. Neurological events reported after COVID-19 vaccines: An analysis of VAERS. *Ann Neurol* 91(6):756–771.

Gargano, J. W., M. Wallace, S. C. Hadler, G. Langley, J. R. Su, M. E. Oster, K. R. Broder, J. Gee, E. Weintraub, T. Shimabukuro, H. M. Scobie, D. Moulia, L. E. Markowitz, M. Wharton, V. V. McNally, J. R. Romero, H. K. Talbot, G. M. Lee, M. F. Daley, and S. E. Oliver. 2021. Use of mRNA COVID-19 vaccine after reports of myocarditis among vaccine recipients: Update from the advisory committee on immunization practices—United States, June 2021. *MMWR Morb Mortal Wkly Rep* 70(27):977–982.

Gee, J. 2024. CDC response to vaccine safety needs for the U.S. COVID-19 vaccination program—an overview of vaccine safety systems. Presentation to the Committee to Review the Centers for Disease Control and Prevention's COVID-19 Vaccine Safety Research and Communications, Washington, DC, August 7.

Gee, J., P. Marquez, J. Su, G. M. Calvert, R. Liu, T. Myers, N. Nair, S. Martin, T. Clark, L. Markowitz, N. Lindsey, B. Zhang, C. Licata, A. Jazwa, M. Sotir, and T. Shimabukuro. 2021. First month of COVID-19 vaccine safety monitoring—United States, December 14, 2020–January 13, 2021. *MMWR Morb Mortal Wkly Rep* 70(8):283–288.

Gee, J., T. T. Shimabukuro, J. R. Su, D. Shay, M. Ryan, S. V. Basavaraju, K. R. Broder, M. Clark, C. Buddy Creech, F. Cunningham, K. Goddard, H. Guy, K. M. Edwards, R. Forshee, T. Hamburger, A. M. Hause, N. P. Klein, I. Kracalik, C. Lamer, D. A. Loran, M. M. McNeil, J. Montgomery, P. Moro, T. R. Myers, C. Olson, M. E. Oster, A. J. Sharma, R. Schupbach, E. Weintraub, B. Whitehead, and S. Anderson. 2024. Overview of U.S. COVID-19 vaccine safety surveillance systems. *Vaccine* 42 Suppl 3:125748.

Goddard, K., K. E. Hanson, N. Lewis, E. Weintraub, B. Fireman, and N. P. Klein. 2022a. Incidence of myocarditis/pericarditis following mRNA COVID-19 vaccination among children and younger adults in the United States. *Ann Intern Med* 175(12):1169–1771.

Goddard, K., N. Lewis, B. Fireman, E. Weintraub, T. Shimabukuro, O. Zerbo, T. G. Boyce, M. E. Oster, K. E. Hanson, J. G. Donahue, P. Ross, A. Naleway, J. C. Nelson, B. Lewin, J. M. Glanz, J. T. B. Williams, E. O. Kharbanda, W. Katherine Yih, and N. P. Klein. 2022b. Risk of myocarditis and pericarditis following BNT162b2 and mRNA-1273 COVID-19 vaccination. *Vaccine* 40(35):5153–5159.

Greinacher, A., T. Thiele, T. E. Warkentin, K. Weisser, P. A. Kyrle, and S. Eichinger. 2021. Thrombotic thrombocytopenia after ChAdOx1 nCOV-19 vaccination. *N Engl J Med* 384(22):2092–2101.

Haendel, M. A., C. G. Chute, T. D. Bennett, D. A. Eichmann, J. Guinney, W. A. Kibbe, P. R. O. Payne, E. R. Pfaff, P. N. Robinson, J. H. Saltz, H. Spratt, C. Suver, J. Wilbanks, A. B. Wilcox, A. E. Williams, C. Wu, C. Blacketer, R. L. Bradford, J. J. Cimino, M. Clark, E. W. Colmenares, P. A. Francis, D. Gabriel, A. Graves, R. Hemadri, S. S. Hong, G. Hripscak, D. Jiao, J. G. Klann, K. Kostka, A. M. Lee, H. P. Lehmann, L. Lingrey, R. T. Miller, M. Morris, S. N. Murphy, K. Natarajan, M. B. Palchuk, U. Sheikh, H. Solbrig, S. Visweswaran, A. Walden, K. M. Walters, G. M. Weber, X. T. Zhang, R. L. Zhu, B. Amor, A. T. Girvin, A. Manna, N. Qureshi, M. G. Kurilla, S. G. Michael, L. M. Portilla, J. L. Rutter, C. P. Austin, K. R. Gersing, and N. C. Consortium. 2021. The National COVID Cohort Collaborative (N3C): Rationale, design, infrastructure, and deployment. *J Am Med Inform Assoc* 28(3):427–443.

Hanson, K. E., K. Goddard, N. Lewis, B. Fireman, T. R. Myers, N. Bakshi, E. Weintraub, J. G. Donahue, J. C. Nelson, S. Xu, J. M. Glanz, J. T. B. Williams, J. D. Alpern, and N. P. Klein. 2022. Incidence of Guillain-Barre Syndrome after COVID-19 vaccination in the vaccine safety datalink. *JAMA Netw Open* 5(4):e228879.

Hause, A. M., J. Baggs, P. Marquez, T. R. Myers, J. R. Su, P. G. Blanc, J. A. Gwira Baumblatt, E. J. Woo, J. Gee, T. T. Shimabukuro, and D. K. Shay. 2022a. Safety monitoring of COVID-19 vaccine booster doses among adults—United States, September 22, 2021–February 6, 2022. *MMWR Morb Mortal Wkly Rep* 71(7):249–254.

Hause, A. M., J. Gee, T. Johnson, A. Jazwa, P. Marquez, E. Miller, J. Su, T. T. Shimabukuro, and D. K. Shay. 2021. Anxiety-related adverse event clusters after Janssen COVID-19 vaccination - five U.S. mass vaccination sites, April 2021. *MMWR Morb Mortal Wkly Rep* 70(18):685–688.

Hause, A. M., P. Marquez, B. Zhang, T. R. Myers, J. Gee, J. R. Su, P. G. Blanc, A. Thomas, D. Thompson, T. T. Shimabukuro, and D. K. Shay. 2022b. Safety monitoring of bivalent COVID-19 mRNA vaccine booster doses among persons aged >/=12 years—United States, August 31–October 23, 2022. *MMWR Morb Mortal Wkly Rep* 71(44):1401–1406.

Hause, A. M., P. Marquez, B. Zhang, J. R. Su, T. R. Myers, J. Gee, S. S. Panchanathan, D. Thompson, T. T. Shimabukuro, and D. K. Shay. 2023. Safety monitoring of bivalent COVID-19 mRNA vaccine booster doses among children aged 5–11 years—United States, October 12–January 1, 2023. *MMWR Morb Mortal Wkly Rep* 72(2):39–43.

Hause, A. M., B. Zhang, X. Yue, P. Marquez, T. R. Myers, C. Parker, J. Gee, J. Su, T. T. Shimabukuro, and D. K. Shay. 2022c. Reactogenicity of simultaneous COVID-19 mRNA booster and influenza vaccination in the US. *JAMA Netw Open* 5(7):e2222241.

HHS (Department of Health and Human Services). 2024. VAERS data use guide. https://vaers.hhs.gov/data/dataguide.html (accessed August 7, 2025).

Hickey, K. 2025. *The PREP Act and COVID-19, part 2: The PREP Act declaration for COVID-19 countermeasures.* Library of Congress, Congressional Research Service. https://www.congress.gov/crs-product/LSB10730 (accessed August 7, 2025).

Kachikis, A., J. A. Englund, M. Singleton, I. Covelli, A. L. Drake, and L. O. Eckert. 2021. Short-term reactions among pregnant and lactating individuals in the first wave of the COVID-19 vaccine rollout. *JAMA Netw Open* 4(8):e2121310.

Katherine Yih, W., M. F. Daley, J. Duffy, B. Fireman, D. McClure, J. Nelson, L. Qian, N. Smith, G. Vazquez-Benitez, E. Weintraub, J. T. B. Williams, S. Xu, and J. C. Maro. 2023. Tree-based data mining for safety assessment of first COVID-19 booster doses in the vaccine safety datalink. *Vaccine* 41(2):460–466.

Kenigsberg, T. A., K. Goddard, K. E. Hanson, N. Lewis, N. Klein, S. A. Irving, A. L. Naleway, B. Crane, T. L. Kauffman, S. Xu, M. F. Daley, L. P. Hurley, R. Kaiser, L. A. Jackson, A. Jazwa, and E. S. Weintraub. 2023a. Simultaneous administration of mRNA COVID-19 bivalent booster and influenza vaccines. *Vaccine* 41(39):5678–5682.

Kenigsberg, T. A., K. E. Hanson, N. P. Klein, O. Zerbo, K. Goddard, S. Xu, W. K. Yih, S. A. Irving, L. P. Hurley, J. M. Glanz, R. Kaiser, L. A. Jackson, and E. S. Weintraub. 2023b. Safety of simultaneous vaccination with COVID-19 vaccines in the Vaccine Safety Datalink. *Vaccine* 41(32):4658–4665.

Klein, N. 2021. Rapid cycle analysis to monitor the safety of COVID-19 vaccines in near real-time within the vaccine safety datalink: Myocarditis and anaphylaxis. Paper read at Vaccine Safety Datalink – Immunization Safety Office, CDC: Atlanta, GA.

Klein, N. P., N. Lewis, K. Goddard, B. Fireman, O. Zerbo, K. E. Hanson, J. G. Donahue, E. O. Kharbanda, A. Naleway, J. C. Nelson, S. Xu, W. K. Yih, J. M. Glanz, J. T. B. Williams, S. J. Hambidge, B. J. Lewin, T. T. Shimabukuro, F. DeStefano, and E. S. Weintraub. 2021. Surveillance for adverse events after COVID-19 mRNA vaccination. *JAMA* 326(14):1390–1399.

Korinthenberg, R., and J. J. Sejvar. 2020. The brighton collaboration case definition: Comparison in a retrospective and prospective cohort of children with Guillain-Barre Syndrome. *J Peripher Nerv Syst* 25(4):344–349.

Lee, G. M. 2021. COVID-19 vaccine safety technical (vast) subgroup. Atlanta, GA. https://stacks.cdc.gov/view/cdc/107716 (accessed January 23, 2025).

Lee, G. M., and R. Hopkins. 2021. COVID-19 vaccine safety technical (vast) subgroup: Discussion and interpretation, Atlanta, GA.

Lipkind, H. S., G. Vazquez-Benitez, M. DeSilva, K. K. Vesco, C. Ackerman-Banks, J. Zhu, T. G. Boyce, M. F. Daley, C. C. Fuller, D. Getahun, S. A. Irving, L. A. Jackson, J. T. B. Williams, O. Zerbo, M. M. McNeil, C. K. Olson, E. Weintraub, and E. O. Kharbanda. 2022. Receipt of COVID-19 vaccine during pregnancy and preterm or small-for-gestational-age at birth-eight integrated health care organizations, United States, December 15, 2020–July 22, 2021. *MMWR Morb Mortal Wkly Rep* 71(1):26–30.

MacNeil, J. R., J. R. Su, K. R. Broder, A. Y. Guh, J. W. Gargano, M. Wallace, S. C. Hadler, H. M. Scobie, A. E. Blain, D. Moulia, M. F. Daley, V. V. McNally, J. R. Romero, H. K. Talbot, G. M. Lee, B. P. Bell, and S. E. Oliver. 2021. Updated recommendations from the Advisory Committee on Immunization Practices for use of the Janssen (Johnson & Johnson) COVID-19 vaccine after reports of thrombosis with thrombocytopenia syndrome among vaccine recipients—United States, April 2021. *MMWR Morb Mortal Wkly Rep* 70(17):651–656.

Madni, S. A., A. J. Sharma, L. H. Zauche, A. V. Waters, J. F. Nahabedian, 3rd, T. Johnson, C. K. Olson, and CDC COVID-19 Vaccine Pregnancy Registry Work Group. 2024. CDC COVID-19 vaccine pregnancy registry: Design, data collection, response rates, and cohort description. *Vaccine* 42(7):1469–1477.

Markowitz, L. E., R. H. Hopkins, Jr., K. R. Broder, G. M. Lee, K. M. Edwards, M. F. Daley, L. A. Jackson, J. C. Nelson, L. E. Riley, V. V. McNally, R. Schechter, P. N. Whitley-Williams, F. Cunningham, M. Clark, M. Ryan, K. M. Farizo, H. L. Wong, J. Kelman, T. Beresnev, V. Marshall, D. K. Shay, J. Gee, J. Woo, M. M. McNeil, J. R. Su, T. T. Shimabukuro, M. Wharton, and H. Keipp Talbot. 2024. COVID-19 vaccine safety technical (vast) work group: Enhancing vaccine safety monitoring during the pandemic. *Vaccine* 42(Suppl 3):125549.

Marschner, C. A., K. E. Shaw, F. S. Tijmes, M. Fronza, S. Khullar, M. A. Seidman, P. Thavendiranathan, J. A. Udell, R. M. Wald, and K. Hanneman. 2023. Myocarditis following COVID-19 vaccination. *Heart Fail Clin* 19(2):251–264.

McNeil, M. M., J. Gee, E. S. Weintraub, E. A. Belongia, G. M. Lee, J. M. Glanz, J. D. Nordin, N. P. Klein, R. Baxter, A. L. Naleway, L. A. Jackson, S. B. Omer, S. J. Jacobsen, and F. DeStefano. 2014. The vaccine safety datalink: Successes and challenges monitoring vaccine safety. *Vaccine* 32(42):5390–5398.

Montgomery, J., M. Ryan, R. Engler, D. Hoffman, B. McClenathan, L. Collins, D. Loran, D. Hrncir, K. Herring, M. Platzer, N. Adams, A. Sanou, and L. T. Cooper, Jr. 2021. Myocarditis following immunization with mRNA COVID-19 vaccines in members of the US military. *JAMA Cardiol* 6(10):1202–1206.

Morgan, H. J., H. J. Clothier, G. Sepulveda Kattan, J. H. Boyd, and J. P. Buttery. 2024. Acute disseminated encephalomyelitis and transverse myelitis following COVID-19 vaccination: A self-controlled case series analysis. *Vaccine* 42(9):2212–2219.

Moro, P. L., G. Carlock, N. Fifadara, T. Habenicht, B. Zhang, P. Strid, and P. Marquez. 2024. Safety monitoring of bivalent mRNA COVID-19 vaccine among pregnant persons in the vaccine adverse event reporting system—United States, September 1, 2022–March 31, 2023. *Vaccine* 42(9):2380–2384.

Moro, P. L., P. Haber, and M. M. McNeil. 2019. Challenges in evaluating post-licensure vaccine safety: Observations from the Centers for Disease Control and Prevention. *Expert Rev Vaccines* 18(10):1091–1101.

Moro, P. L., L. Panagiotakopoulos, T. Oduyebo, C. K. Olson, and T. Myers. 2021. Monitoring the safety of COVID-19 vaccines in pregnancy in the US. *Hum Vaccin Immunother* 17(12):4705–4713.

Myers, T. R., P. L. Marquez, J. M. Gee, A. M. Hause, L. Panagiotakopoulos, B. Zhang, I. McCullum, C. Licata, C. K. Olson, S. Rahman, S. B. Kennedy, M. Cardozo, C. R. Patel, L. Maxwell, J. R. Kallman, D. K. Shay, and T. T. Shimabukuro. 2023. The V-safe after vaccination health checker: Active vaccine safety monitoring during CDC's COVID-19 pandemic response. *Vaccine* 41(7):1310–1318.

Nasreen, S., Y. Jiang, H. Lu, A. Lee, C. L. Cutland, A. Gentile, N. Giglio, K. Macartney, L. Deng, B. Liu, N. Sonneveld, K. Bellamy, H. J. Clothier, G. Sepulveda Kattan, M. Naus, Z. Naveed, N. Z. Janjua, L. Nguyen, A. Hviid, E. Poukka, J. Perala, T. Leino, L. A. Chandra, J. A. Thobari, B. J. Park, N. K. Choi, N. Y. Jeong, S. A. Madhi, F. Villalobos, M. Solorzano, C. A. Bissacco, J. J. Carreras-Martinez, E. Correcher-Martinez, A. Urchueguia-Fornes, D. Roy, A. Yeomans, T. Aurelius, K. Morton, G. Di Mauro, M. C. Sturkenboom, J. J. Sejvar, K. A. Top, K. Batty, L. Ghebreab, J. B. Griffin, H. Petousis-Harris, J. Buttery, S. Black, and J. C. Kwong. 2025. Risk of Guillain-Barre Syndrome after COVID-19 vaccination or SARS-CoV-2 infection: A multinational self-controlled case series study. *Vaccine* 60:127291.

Oliver, S. E., J. W. Gargano, M. Marin, M. Wallace, K. G. Curran, M. Chamberland, N. McClung, D. Campos-Outcalt, R. L. Morgan, S. Mbaeyi, J. R. Romero, H. K. Talbot, G. M. Lee, B. P. Bell, and K. Dooling. 2020. The Advisory Committee on Immunization Practices' interim recommendation for use of Pfizer-BioNTech COVID-19 vaccine—United States, December 2020. *MMWR Morb Mortal Wkly Rep* 69(50):1922–1924.

Oliver, S. E., M. Wallace, I. See, S. Mbaeyi, M. Godfrey, S. C. Hadler, T. C. Jatlaoui, E. Twentyman, M. M. Hughes, A. K. Rao, A. Fiore, J. R. Su, K. R. Broder, T. Shimabukuro, A. Lale, D. K. Shay, L. E. Markowitz, M. Wharton, B. P. Bell, O. Brooks, V. McNally, G. M. Lee, H. K. Talbot, and M. F. Daley. 2022. Use of the Janssen (Johnson & Johnson) COVID-19 vaccine: Updated interim recommendations from the Advisory Committee on Immunization Practices - United States, December 2021. *MMWR Morb Mortal Wkly Rep* 71(3):90–95.

Oster, M. E., D. K. Shay, J. R. Su, J. Gee, C. B. Creech, K. R. Broder, K. Edwards, J. H. Soslow, J. M. Dendy, E. Schlaudecker, S. M. Lang, E. D. Barnett, F. L. Ruberg, M. J. Smith, M. J. Campbell, R. D. Lopes, L. S. Sperling, J. A. Baumblatt, D. L. Thompson, P. L. Marquez, P. Strid, J. Woo, R. Pugsley, S. Reagan-Steiner, F. DeStefano, and T. T. Shimabukuro. 2022. Myocarditis cases reported after mRNA-based COVID-19 vaccination in the US from December 2020 to August 2021. *JAMA* 327(4):331–340.

Petersen, I., I. Douglas, and H. Whitaker. 2016. Self controlled case series methods: An alternative to standard epidemiological study designs. *BMJ* 354:i4515.

Phillips, A., Y. Jiang, D. Walsh, N. Andrews, M. Artama, H. Clothier, L. Cullen, L. Deng, S. Escolano, A. Gentile, G. Gidding, N. Giglio, T. Junker, W. Huang, N. Janjua, J. Kwong, J. Li, S. Nasreen, M. Naus, Z. Naveed, A. Pillsbury, J. Stowe, T. Vo, J. Buttery, H. Petousis-Harris, S. Black, and A. Hviid. 2023. Background rates of adverse events of special interest for COVID-19 vaccines: A Multinational Global Vaccine Data Network (GVDN) analysis. *Vaccine* 41(42):6227–6238.

Polack, F. P., S. J. Thomas, N. Kitchin, J. Absalon, A. Gurtman, S. Lockhart, J. L. Perez, G. Perez Marc, E. D. Moreira, C. Zerbini, R. Bailey, K. A. Swanson, S. Roychoudhury, K. Koury, P. Li, W. V. Kalina, D. Cooper, R. W. Frenck, Jr., L. L. Hammitt, O. Tureci, H. Nell, A. Schaefer, S. Unal, D. B. Tresnan, S. Mather, P. R. Dormitzer, U. Sahin, K. U. Jansen, W. C. Gruber, and C4591001 Clinical Trial Group. 2020. Safety and efficacy of the BNT162b2 mRNA COVID-19 vaccine. *N Engl J Med* 383(27):2603–2615.

Razen, S. 2021. Public comment at CDC ACIP April 23, 2021 meeting (starting at 30:35). https://www.youtube.com/watch?v=j5KqOLNpTt4&list=PLvrp9iOILTQb6D9e1YZWpbUvzfptNMKx2&index=51 (accessed August 25, 2025).

Rosenblum, H. G., J. Gee, R. Liu, P. L. Marquez, B. Zhang, P. Strid, W. E. Abara, M. M. McNeil, T. R. Myers, A. M. Hause, J. R. Su, L. E. Markowitz, T. T. Shimabukuro, and D. K. Shay. 2022. Safety of mRNA vaccines administered during the initial 6 months of the US COVID-19 vaccination programme: An observational study of reports to the Vaccine Adverse Event Reporting System and V-safe. *Lancet Infect Dis* 22(6):802–812.

Rosenblum, H. G., S. C. Hadler, D. Moulia, T. T. Shimabukuro, J. R. Su, N. K. Tepper, K. C. Ess, E. J. Woo, A. Mba-Jonas, M. Alimchandani, N. Nair, N. P. Klein, K. E. Hanson, L. E. Markowitz, M. Wharton, V. V. McNally, J. R. Romero, H. K. Talbot, G. M. Lee, M. F. Daley, S. A. Mbaeyi, and S. E. Oliver. 2021. Use of COVID-19 vaccines after reports of adverse events among adult recipients of Janssen (Johnson & Johnson) and mRNA COVID-19 vaccines (Pfizer-BioNTech and Moderna): Update from the Advisory Committee on Immunization Practices—United States, July 2021. *MMWR Morb Mortal Wkly Rep* 70(32):1094–1099.

Sakaeda, T., A. Tamon, K. Kadoyama, and Y. Okuno. 2013. Data mining of the public version of the FDA adverse event reporting system. *Int J Med Sci* 10(7):796–803.

Salmon, D., D. J. Opel, M. Z. Dudley, J. Brewer, and R. Breiman. 2021. Reflections on governance, communication, and equity: Challenges and opportunities in COVID-19 vaccination. *Health Aff (Millwood)* 40(3):419–425.

See, I. 2021. Updates on thrombosis with thrombocytopenia syndrome (TTS). Paper read at Advisory Committee on Immunization Practices (ACIP) meeting, December 16, Atlanta, GA.

See, I., A. Lale, P. Marquez, M. B. Streiff, A. P. Wheeler, N. K. Tepper, E. J. Woo, K. R. Broder, K. M. Edwards, R. Gallego, A. I. Geller, K. A. Jackson, S. Sharma, K. R. Talaat, E. B. Walter, I. J. Akpan, T. L. Ortel, V. C. Urrutia, S. C. Walker, J. C. Yui, T. T. Shimabukuro, A. Mba-Jonas, J. R. Su, and D. K. Shay. 2022. Case series of thrombosis with thrombocytopenia syndrome after COVID-19 vaccination—United States, December 2020 to August 2021. *Ann Intern Med* 175(4):513–522.

See, I., J. R. Su, A. Lale, E. J. Woo, A. Y. Guh, T. T. Shimabukuro, M. B. Streiff, A. K. Rao, A. P. Wheeler, S. F. Beavers, A. P. Durbin, K. Edwards, E. Miller, T. A. Harrington, A. Mba-Jonas, N. Nair, D. T. Nguyen, K. R. Talaat, V. C. Urrutia, S. C. Walker, C. B. Creech, T. A. Clark, F. DeStefano, and K. R. Broder. 2021. US case reports of cerebral venous sinus thrombosis with thrombocytopenia after Ad26.COV2.S vaccination, March 2 to April 21, 2021. *JAMA* 325(24):2448–2456.

Sejvar, J. J., K. S. Kohl, J. Gidudu, A. Amato, N. Bakshi, R. Baxter, D. R. Burwen, D. R. Cornblath, J. Cleerbout, K. M. Edwards, U. Heininger, R. Hughes, N. Khuri-Bulos, R. Korinthenberg, B. J. Law, U. Munro, H. C. Maltezou, P. Nell, J. Oleske, R. Sparks, P. Velentgas, P. Vermeer, M. Wiznitzer, and Brighton Collaboration GBS Working Group. 2011. Guillain-Barre Syndrome and Fisher Syndrome: Case definitions and guidelines for collection, analysis, and presentation of immunization safety data. *Vaccine* 29(3):599–612.

Shay, D. K., J. Gee, J. R. Su, T. R. Myers, P. Marquez, R. Liu, B. Zhang, C. Licata, T. A. Clark, and T. T. Shimabukuro. 2021. Safety monitoring of the Janssen (Johnson & Johnson) COVID-19 vaccine—United States, March–April 2021. *MMWR Morb Mortal Wkly Rep* 70(18):680–684.

Shimabukuro, T. 2021a. Allergic reactions including anaphylaxis after receipt of the first dose of Moderna COVID-19 vaccine—United States, December 21, 2020–January 10, 2021. *Am J Transplant* 21(3):1326–1331.

Shimabukuro, T. T. 2021b. Thrombosis with thrombocytopenia syndrome (TTS) following Janssen COVID-19 vaccine, April 23. Atlanta, GA. https://stacks.cdc.gov/view/cdc/107508 (accessed August 25, 2025).

Shimabukuro, T. 2022. Update on myocarditis following mRNA COVID-19 vaccination. Paper read at Vaccines and Related Biological Products Advisory Committee (VRBPAC), June 14, Silver Spring, MD.

Shimabukuro, T. T. 2023a. COVID-19 mRNA bivalent booster vaccine safety. Paper read at Advisory Committee on Immunization Practices (ACIP) meeting, February 24, Atlanta, GA.

Shimabukuro, T. T. 2023b. Update: V-safe after vaccination health checker. Paper read at Advisory Committee on Immunization Practices (ACIP) meeting, April 19, Atlanta, GA.

Shimabukuro, T. T., M. Cole, and J. R. Su. 2021a. Reports of anaphylaxis after receipt of mRNA COVID-19 vaccines in the US—December 14, 2020–January 18, 2021. *JAMA* 325(11):1101–1102.

Shimabukuro, T. T., S. Y. Kim, T. R. Myers, P. L. Moro, T. Oduyebo, L. Panagiotakopoulos, P. L. Marquez, C. K. Olson, R. Liu, K. T. Chang, S. R. Ellington, V. K. Burkel, A. N. Smoots, C. J. Green, C. Licata, B. C. Zhang, M. Alimchandani, A. Mba-Jonas, S. W. Martin, J. M. Gee, D. M. Meaney-Delman, and CDC V-safe COVID-19 Pregnancy Registry Team. 2021b. Preliminary findings of mRNA COVID-19 vaccine safety in pregnant persons. *N Engl J Med* 384(24):2273–2282.

Shimabukuro, T. T., and N. Klein. 2023. COVID-19 mRNA bivalent booster vaccine safety. Paper read at Vaccines and Related Biological Products Advisory Committee meeting, January 26, Silver Spring, MD.

Shimabukuro, T. T., M. Nguyen, D. Martin, and F. DeStefano. 2015. Safety monitoring in the Vaccine Adverse Event Reporting System (VAERS). *Vaccine* 33(36):4398–4405.

U.S. GAO (Government Accountability Office). 2021. *Covid-19: Critical vaccine distribution, supply chain, program integrity, and other challenges require focused federal attention.* U.S. Government Accountability Office.

Varricchio, F., J. Iskander, F. Destefano, R. Ball, R. Pless, M. M. Braun, and R. T. Chen. 2004. Understanding vaccine safety information from the Vaccine Adverse Event Reporting System. *Pediatr Infect Dis J* 23(4):287–294.

Wallace, M., D. Moulia, A. E. Blain, E. K. Ricketts, F. S. Minhaj, R. Link-Gelles, K. G. Curran, S. C. Hadler, A. Asif, M. Godfrey, E. Hall, A. Fiore, S. Meyer, J. R. Su, E. Weintraub, M. E. Oster, T. T. Shimabukuro, D. Campos-Outcalt, R. L. Morgan, B. P. Bell, O. Brooks, H. K. Talbot, G. M. Lee, M. F. Daley, and S. E. Oliver. 2022. The Advisory Committee on Immunization Practices' recommendation for use of Moderna COVID-19 vaccine in adults aged >/=18 years and considerations for extended intervals for administration of primary series doses of mRNA COVID-19 vaccines—United States, February 2022. *MMWR Morb Mortal Wkly Rep* 71(11):416–421.

Williams, S. E., N. P. Klein, N. Halsey, C. L. Dekker, R. P. Baxter, C. D. Marchant, P. S. LaRussa, R. C. Sparks, J. I. Tokars, B. A. Pahud, L. Aukes, K. Jakob, S. Coronel, H. Choi, B. A. Slade, and K. M. Edwards. 2011. Overview of the clinical consult case review of adverse events following immunization: Clinical Immunization Safety Assessment (CISA) network 2004–2009. *Vaccine* 29(40):6920–6927.

Wong, H. L., E. Tworkoski, C. Ke Zhou, M. Hu, D. Thompson, B. Lufkin, R. Do, L. Feinberg, Y. Chillarige, R. Dimova, P. C. Lloyd, T. MaCurdy, R. A. Forshee, J. A. Kelman, A. Shoaibi, and S. A. Anderson. 2023. Surveillance of COVID-19 vaccine safety among elderly persons aged 65 years and older. *Vaccine* 41(2):532–539.

Wong, K. K., C. M. Heilig, A. Hause, T. R. Myers, C. K. Olson, J. Gee, P. Marquez, P. Strid, and D. K. Shay. 2022. Menstrual irregularities and vaginal bleeding after COVID-19 vaccination reported to V-safe active surveillance, USA in December, 2020–January, 2022: An observational cohort study. *Lancet Digit Health* 4(9):e667–e675.

Woo, E. J., A. Mba-Jonas, R. B. Dimova, M. Alimchandani, C. E. Zinderman, and N. Nair. 2021. Association of receipt of the Ad26.COV2.S COVID-19 vaccine with presumptive Guillain-Barre Syndrome, February–July 2021. *JAMA* 326(16):1606–1613.

Xu, S., R. Huang, L. S. Sy, S. C. Glenn, D. S. Ryan, K. Morrissette, D. K. Shay, G. Vazquez-Benitez, J. M. Glanz, N. P. Klein, D. McClure, E. G. Liles, E. S. Weintraub, H. F. Tseng, and L. Qian. 2021. COVID-19 vaccination and non-COVID-19 mortality risk - seven integrated health care organizations, United States, December 14, 2020–July 31, 2021. *MMWR Morb Mortal Wkly Rep* 70(43):1520–1524.

Xu, S., R. Huang, L. S. Sy, V. Hong, S. C. Glenn, D. S. Ryan, K. Morrissette, G. Vazquez-Benitez, J. M. Glanz, N. P. Klein, B. Fireman, D. McClure, E. G. Liles, E. S. Weintraub, H. F. Tseng, and L. Qian. 2023. A safety study evaluating non-change to COVID-19 mortality risk following COVID-19 vaccination. *Vaccine* 41(3):844–854.

Xu, S., L. S. Sy, V. Hong, P. Farrington, S. C. Glenn, D. S. Ryan, A. M. Shirley, B. J. Lewin, H. F. Tseng, G. Vazquez-Benitez, J. M. Glanz, B. Fireman, D. L. McClure, L. P. Hurley, O. Yu, M. Wernecke, N. Smith, E. S. Weintraub, and L. Qian. 2024. Mortality risk after COVID-19 vaccination: A self-controlled case series study. *Vaccine* 42(7):1731–1737.

Yih, W. K., M. F. Daley, J. Duffy, B. Fireman, D. McClure, J. Nelson, L. Qian, N. Smith, G. Vazquez-Benitez, E. Weintraub, J. T. B. Williams, S. Xu, and J. C. Maro. 2023. A broad assessment of COVID-19 vaccine safety using tree-based data-mining in the vaccine safety datalink. *Vaccine* 41(3):826–835.

Yih, W. K., J. Duffy, J. R. Su, S. Bazel, B. Fireman, L. Hurley, J. C. Maro, P. Marquez, P. Moro, N. Nair, J. Nelson, N. Smith, M. Sundaram, G. Vasquez-Benitez, E. Weintraub, S. Xu, and T. Shimabukuro. 2024. Tinnitus after COVID-19 vaccination: Findings from the Vaccine Adverse Event Reporting System and the Vaccine Safety Datalink. *Am J Otolaryngol* 45(6):104448.

Yousaf, A. R., M. M. Cortese, A. W. Taylor, K. R. Broder, M. E. Oster, J. M. Wong, A. Y. Guh, D. W. McCormick, S. Kamidani, E. P. Schlaudecker, K. M. Edwards, C. B. Creech, M. A. Staat, E. D. Belay, P. Marquez, J. R. Su, M. B. Salzman, D. Thompson, A. P. Campbell, and MIS-C Investigation Authorship Group. 2022. Reported cases of multisystem inflammatory syndrome in children aged 12–20 years in the USA who received a COVID-19 vaccine, December, 2020, through August, 2021: A surveillance investigation. *Lancet Child Adolesc Health* 6(5):303–312.

Zauche, L. H., B. Wallace, A. N. Smoots, C. K. Olson, T. Oduyebo, S. Y. Kim, E. E. Petersen, J. Ju, J. Beauregard, A. J. Wilcox, C. E. Rose, D. M. Meaney-Delman, S. R. Ellington, for the CDC V-safe COVID-19 Pregnancy Registry Team. 2021. Receipt of mRNA COVID-19 vaccines and risk of spontaneous abortion. *N Engl J Med* 385(16):1533–1535.

Zhou, Z. H., M. M. Cortese, J. L. Fang, R. Wood, D. S. Hummell, K. A. Risma, A. E. Norton, M. KuKuruga, S. Kirshner, R. L. Rabin, C. Agarabi, M. A. Staat, N. Halasa, R. E. Ware, A. Stahl, M. McMahon, P. Browning, P. Maniatis, S. Bolcen, K. M. Edwards, J. R. Su, S. Dharmarajan, R. Forshee, K. R. Broder, S. Anderson, and S. Kozlowski. 2023. Evaluation of association of anti-PEG antibodies with anaphylaxis after mRNA COVID-19 vaccination. *Vaccine* 41(28):4183–4189.

Zou, C., X. Xue, and J. Qian. 2022. Characteristics and comparison of adverse events of coronavirus disease 2019 vaccines reported to the United States Vaccine Adverse Event Reporting System between 14 December 2020 and 8 October 2021. *Front Med (Lausanne)* 9:826327.

3

Communications

PUBLIC HEALTH COMMUNICATIONS

Sound, evidence-based information is essential when it comes to fostering health care providers, patient, and public understanding and behavior about the benefits, risks, and value of public health recommendations. However, as the recent COVID pandemic made clear, multiple complexities and challenges exist in providing health and medical information, particularly if the goals include health care provider (HCP) endorsement of recommendations. Increased vaccine uptake to prevent disease is typically a goal of vaccination and related risk–benefit information and communication. It is also often assumed that achieving outcomes such as these with public health recommendations is primarily a matter of repeatedly and visibly providing "clear" (e.g., easily understood), "consistent" (e.g. uniform or unchanging), and "tailored" (e.g., customized) risk–benefit information and messages via "trusted" messengers using an array of traditional, social, and digital media channels and platforms (French et al., 2020).

While this assumption underlies fundamental concepts in health communication, its simplicity is deceptive. Much ultimately impacts public health entities' and government agencies' ability to act these concepts, and many factors influence the ability to deliver on these. Most public health programs and agencies, for instance, lack the financial and other resources needed to create and support communication programs that can continually and visibly reach multiple target subpopulations with customized information (Nowak et al., 2015). Furthermore, to the extent that information and recommendations do reach them, a host of factors, ranging from varying levels of trust in those providing information and advice to differences in health, science, and reading literacy and ability to undertake recommended actions, significantly affect risk–benefit perceptions, health decision making, and behaviors.

In medicine and public health (as cases and outbreaks of COVID, Ebola, and Mpox viruses showed), it is particularly difficult to effectively communicate (e.g., provide clear, consistent, and easily understandable information) when the situation involves evolving scientific knowledge about new or emerging infectious disease; emergently authorized or newly licensed vaccines; false and misleading information; and evolving vaccination recommendations based on updated scientific knowledge. New and emerging infectious diseases bring uncertainties regarding transmission, severity and consequences of illness, and susceptibility (including which subpopulations and individuals are most vulnerable to infection, severe illness, and death) and differing projections regarding how fast and far infections and disease will spread. Those requiring recently authorized and licensed vaccines bring additional communication challenges related to the uncertainties regarding their efficacy and effectiveness (e.g., ability to protect against infection and/or severe disease and death), durability of protection, and safety, including immediate and short-term reactions to short- and long-term rare but serious adverse events (AEs). These challenges were compounded during the COVID pandemic by the use of Emergency Use Authorizations (EUAs), a regulatory mechanism unfamiliar to much of the public, which made it more difficult to communicate evolving evidence and may have contributed to confusion or mistrust regarding the vaccines' safety and approval status.

As an example, EUAs enable the Food and Drug Administration (FDA) to permit the use of not yet licensed medical products, such as vaccines, when no adequate alternatives (e.g., a licensed vaccine) are available. FDA issued EUAs in December 2020 for the Pfizer/BioNTech and Moderna mRNA COVID vaccines based on clinical trial data that indicated the known and potential benefits outweighed the known and potential risks. Since EUAs had not been used to make new vaccines quickly and more widely available in a pandemic, this created additional communication challenges (Hammershaimb et al., 2022). As relatively few HCPs, people for whom the vaccines were recommended, and the broader public were familiar with the EUA process, much information regarding the safety, efficacy, and benefits needed to be continuously provided and updated to foster understanding of vaccination recommendations and address questions or concerns that had given rise to hesitancy. In addition, concerns about vaccines' novelty (e.g., mRNA technology) and safety (e.g., immediate reactions, long-term side effects), trust in authorities (e.g., science, public health, elected officials, HCPs), misleading information, and beliefs about susceptibility and likelihood of severe illness heightened reluctance.

VACCINE AND VACCINATION-RELATED BENEFIT–RISK COMMUNICATION

The understanding of effects (both intended and unintended), and effectiveness of vaccine and vaccination-related benefit–risk communication are influenced by uncertainties involving the recommended vaccine(s) and the disease. First, how well recommendations, particularly ones involving newly developed and recommended vaccines, are perceived as individually beneficial is shaped by a host of considerations. These include perceptions regarding how well the vaccine can prevent or mitigate disease, particularly serious illness and death, and whether it may also reduce transmission (e.g., can it prevent infection and/or significantly impede human-to-human transmission); actual or expected efficacy in preventing infection and/or serious illness and protecting individuals and subpopulations most susceptible to severe illness; available evidence or data regarding immediate, short-term, and longer-term reactions (e.g., type and prevalence in the days after vaccination); and whether the vaccine is safer and more effective than alternatives (e.g., treatments, natural infection). Furthermore, perceptions of COVID vaccines and vaccination recommendations were also influenced by early and robust uptake by those at highest risk of harm, corroborated and uncorroborated reports of serious AEs (e.g., myocarditis in male young adults after mRNA vaccination), revisions and expansion of recommendations (e.g., to encompass more people, to include children) and vaccine refinements (e.g., to protect against new strains). As was seen during the pandemic, changing and broadening vaccination recommendations can engender concern, questions, doubts, and skepticism among individuals who have medical conditions that put them at elevated risk for severe illness and individuals in the broader population who may not perceive the virus to be a significant threat to their health and well-being and/or vaccination to be highly beneficial.

Published research before, during, and after the COVID public health emergency (PHE), including that involving routine recommended childhood and adult vaccines, has identified factors related to vaccine information and communication effects and effectiveness. First, one needs to identify the audience(s) (e.g., who needs to receive risk and benefit information) and articulate the objectives of the information and communication efforts with respect to that audience; that is, what is/are the desired outcomes? For vaccines, potential objectives include widespread or greater awareness and understanding of the benefits and risks, enhanced confidence and/or less hesitancy, or high or increased uptake among people for whom vaccination is recommended. Second, information alone is rarely sufficient for achieving communication and behavioral objectives. Simply providing more information, including that related to vaccine benefits or risks, rarely changes perceptions or motivates uptake (Brewer et al., 2017; Dubé and MacDonald, 2017). Rather, the risk–benefit information needs to have an individual or subpopulation focus (e.g., take into account their knowledge, understanding, concerns, values, and beliefs), well describe the benefits, acknowledge and address barriers to vaccination (e.g., cost, access), and be aligned with people's priorities and decision making (Brewer et al., 2017; Nowak et al., 2017). It has also been found that providing information about both benefits and risks increased trust and fostered vaccination intention, particularly when the HCP was perceived as empathetic and competent (Juanchich et al., 2024). Third, the source or provider of the risk–benefit information matters. Many published studies have documented that immunization providers (e.g., physicians, pediatricians, nurses) are the most trusted source of vaccine and vaccination information (Eller et al., 2019), with high trust associated with vaccination acceptance, including for COVID (Dudley et al., 2022; Warren et al., 2023). It has also been found, including during the pandemic, that media sources, particularly those used because they align with individuals' worldview, affect trust in public health and medical recommendations, and in turn, vaccine-related beliefs and intentions/behavior (Dolman et al., 2023; Sarathchandra and Johnson-Leung, 2024).

People for whom vaccination is recommended are interested in its risks and harms, referred to as "side effects," "adverse reactions," or "adverse events." The inconsistent and varied use of "risk" and "harm," in concert with inconsistent and varied ways to categorize vaccine reactions, presents many communication challenges. "Risk," for instance, can be defined in terms of probability (e.g., the estimated or evidence-based likelihood of a negative outcome), in terms of a known or possible bad outcome (e.g., a very negative or severe outcome being characterized as the risk), or as a synonym for harm (i.e., the bad or severe outcome itself).

Vaccine and immunization safety-related information and communication bring further challenges that affect content and messaging. Many of these challenges stem from the nature of immunization safety data and how they are presented:

- Individual versus population health. Challenges in extrapolating data from population-level benefits/harms to individual risk and vice versa.
- Time required to obtain and analyze valid and reliable data (e.g., medical records), including obtaining adequate sample size for reliable assessment. Rare AEs (e.g., 1 in 100,000) and long-term outcomes (like cancer and autoimmune disorders) require large datasets and time to detect patterns, making confirmation or exclusion of vaccine association difficult.

- The distinction between association and causation. Differentiating what is correlated with versus directly caused by vaccination requires robust study design and analysis.
- Attribution of causality at the individual level (difficulty in objectively showing or knowing whether vaccination prevented infection or severe illness or death). Counterfactuals (non-events) are almost impossible to directly observe for individuals.
- Heterogeneity of risks and benefit/harms balances. Other factors could be associated with, cause, and/or contribute to a significant vaccine reaction or AE (e.g., immune status, age, gender, ethnicity). Identifying and assessing contributing/associated factors takes robust, granular data.
- Moving target. Dynamic likelihood of contracting and/or experiencing severe illness is influenced by vaccination uptake in a community. Risk is not static and changes as more people are vaccinated and the pandemic evolves. Benefits also change.
- Vaccine safety data are complex, and communication is challenging. Data often include risks, ratios, confidence intervals, and statistical estimates, which require translation for public understanding. Many struggle to interpret small probabilities, understand relative versus absolute risk, or contextualize rare events (Reyna et al., 2009; Zipkin et al., 2014).
- Technical versus common language (e.g., side effects, AEs, adverse reactions). Jargon can confuse the public; there's often a gap between scientific and layperson understanding.
- Consensus on findings does not guarantee acceptance or action. Even when data are valid/reliable (e.g., 1 in 25,000 AEs), experts, health professionals, and the public may interpret/recommend different actions. Decision making is influenced by not just data but perceived and personal values of risk, particularly regarding long- versus short-term risks.
- Speculation and misinformation. Unproven fears (e.g., vaccines cause cancer) can be hard to dispel, especially if confirming or disproving such risks is difficult due to the nature of the data.

VACCINE SAFETY COMMUNICATIONS AT THE CENTERS FOR DISEASE CONTROL AND PREVENTION (CDC)

Effective vaccine safety communication depends on having scientifically robust safety data. While benefit–risk communication is essential for informing public health decisions, the role of the Immunization Safety Office (ISO) within CDC is focused specifically on identifying and communicating risks. ISO is charged with collecting, analyzing, and publicly reporting vaccine safety data and identified signals. It does not develop clinical recommendations or policy or integrate benefits and risks; those activities are undertaken by ACIP, the National Center for Immunization and Respiratory Diseases (NCIRD), and other CDC units. By maintaining this separation, ISO preserves the scientific independence of its safety assessments and ensures that its risk evaluations remain analytically distinct from policy development. Vaccine safety communications at CDC are crosscutting; different centers and programs use the information collected from the ISO vaccine safety systems to inform the populations that they serve. Daniel Jernigan, director of the National Center for Emerging Zoonotic and Infectious Diseases,[1] explained to the committee that CDC's vaccine safety communication efforts "are deliberate approaches designed to effectively share accurate, evidence-based information about safety while addressing concerns and building trust in the vaccine safety enterprise" (Jernigan, 2025). This involves being transparent, actively engaging with communities to exchange accurate information, tailoring messages to specific audiences, collaborating with trusted messengers, aligning communication with research and best practices, adapting based on ongoing insights, and combating misinformation (Jernigan, 2025). ISO's statutory remit is to quantify and communicate vaccine-safety risks, not to determine vaccination policy. Public-facing ISO materials therefore focus on reporting numeric risk estimates with appropriate confidence intervals and describing analytic methods, while directing readers to NCIRD and ACIP channels for interpretations that weigh those risks against benefits.[2] Box 3-1 contains examples of CDC's vaccine safety communication efforts, including collaboration between NCIRD and ISO.

CDC targets four key audiences regarding vaccine safety: U.S. federal government agencies, advisory committees, partners and HCPs, and the public. Figure 3-1 contains the various types of communications with each key audience. Federal agencies that monitor vaccine safety signals remain in constant communication, particularly during a PHE or the introduction of a new vaccine. These agencies also hold formal briefings with their advisory committees to coordinate responses. At ACIP meetings—outlined in Chapter 2—ISO staff, vaccine-specific working groups, and—during the PHE—the Vaccine Safety Technical Work Group (VaST) presented findings, which become part of the public record.

To inform HCPs, CDC conducts clinician outreach and communication activity (COCA) calls—subject-matter experts share updates on relevant clinical and public health topics (CDC, 2025a). CDC engages the public through its website, where it posts vaccine-safety-related content. The committee's evaluation of these webpages appears later in this chapter.

---

[1] As of August 28, 2025, Dr. Daniel Jernigan is no longer the director of CDC's NCEZID.
[2] Public Health Service Act, Section 2102, 42nd U.S Congress.

> **BOX 3-1**
> **CDC Vaccine Safety Communication Efforts**
>
> - Vaccine Information Statement
> - Advisory Committees (e.g., Advisory Committee on Immunization Practices)
> - Vaccine guidance for health care providers (HCPs)
> - Domestic HCP and partner training
> - Global HCP and partner training
> - Emergency response
> - Support to state and local health departments
> - Responses to public inquiries
> - Travelers' vaccine guidance
> - Resources for specific populations (e.g., older adults)
> - Immigrant and refugee health guidance
>
> SOURCE: Prepared by the committee and adapted from the presentation by Daniel Jernigan, 2025.

State and territorial public health agencies (SPHAs) were not always treated as core audiences for safety communications during the COVID response. Yet their role as on-the-ground public health implementers requires early, routine, and bidirectional engagement. Conversations with SPHAs should occur on a regular cadence—including just-in-time briefings before major announcements or policy changes—to enable them to act as effective extensions of CDC communication. The absence of consistent coordination early in the pandemic created avoidable confusion and hindered message alignment at the community level (Fraser, 2021).

COMMUNICATIONS DURING THE PHE

During summer 2020, CDC developed a COVID vaccine safety communications strategy in anticipation of vaccine availability (see Figure 3-2) alongside the vaccine development, testing, and authorization timeline; it included identifying key audiences, messages, tactics, trusted messengers, and dissemination channels. Safety monitoring and communication of findings began once vaccines received EUAs and ACIP recommended them (Jernigan, 2025).

Although CDC has various ways of communicating with its partners, not all of them are publicly available or easily accessible. Table 3-1 contains

Federal agencies
(FDA, CMS, VA, DoD, etc.)
- Near daily contact about safety issues
- Formal briefings

Advisory Committees
(CDC ACIP and working groups, FDA VRBPAC, HHS NVAC, HRSA ACCV, WHO GACVS)
- Work group meetings
- Presentations

Partners + Health Care Providers
(Clinicians, state and local health departments, CBOs, professional organizations [e.g., AAP])
- Partner newsletters
- Dear Provider letters
- HCP-focused outlets (e.g., Medscape)
- Guidance/interim clinical considerations/recommendations
- COCA calls
- Trainings
- Website

Public
(General public, special populations [e.g., older adults, travelers, immunocompromised individuals])
- Website
- Vaccine Information Statements
- Social media
- Messages for specific populations (e.g., older adults)
- Videos
- Print materials

FIGURE 3-1 CDC vaccine safety key audiences and communications.
NOTE: AAP = American Academy of Pediatrics; CBO = community-based organization; CDC ACIP = Centers for Disease Control and Prevention Advisory Committee on Immunization Practices; CMS = Centers for Medicare & Medicaid Services; COCA = Clinician Outreach and Communication Activity; DoD = Department of Defense; FDA = Food and Drug Administration; FDA VRBPAC = Food and Drug Administration Vaccines and Related Biological Products Advisory Committee; HCP = health care provider; HHS NVAC = Department of Health and Human Services National Vaccine Advisory Committee; HRSA ACCV = Health Resources and Services Administration Advisory Committee on Childhood Vaccines; VA = Department of Veterans Affairs; WHO GACVS = World Health Organization Global Advisory Committee on Vaccine Safety.
SOURCE: Prepared by the committee and adapted from the presentation by Daniel Jernigan, 2025.

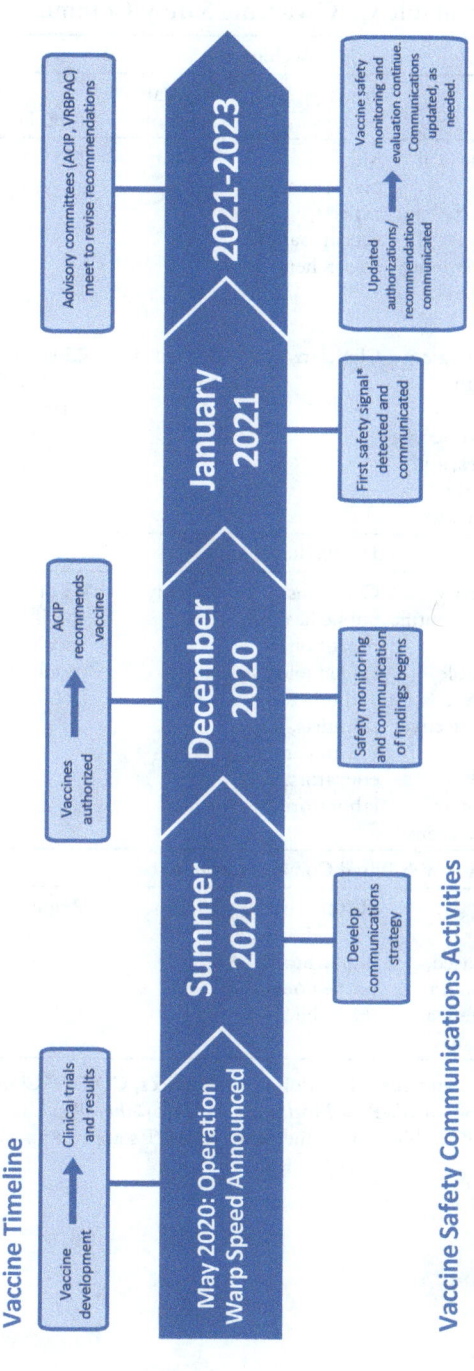

FIGURE 3-2 CDC vaccine safety communication activities timeline during the public health emergency.
NOTE: *Signal: a statistical association found in vaccine safety monitoring; it does not mean there is a true association and requires investigation and evaluation. ACIP = Advisory Committee on Immunization Practices; VRBPAC = Vaccines and Related Biological Products Advisory Committee.
SOURCE: Prepared by the committee and adapted from the presentation by Daniel Jernigan, 2025.

TABLE 3-1 Publicly Available CDC Vaccine Safety Communications

		Meetings/Webinars		
Communication	Purpose	Primary Audience	Regular Schedule	Total During PHE
ACIP Meetings	Convene medical and public health experts who develop recommendations on U.S. use of vaccines	Medical and public health experts, vaccine safety researchers	3x/year	27
COCA Calls	Address emerging public health threats, provide updates on ongoing health issues, and share important clinical guidance	Clinicians	Varied, as needed	23 webinars specific to COVID vaccine safety
		CDC Publications		
MMWR	Be the primary vehicle for scientific publication of timely, reliable, authoritative, accurate, objective, and useful public health information and recommendations	Clinicians, public health practitioners, epidemiologists and other scientists, researchers, educators, and laboratorians	Weekly	43 publications specific to COVID vaccine safety monitoring
		Web-Based Communications		
Webpages	Provide transparent, evidence-based, information on vaccine safety and safety signals	Health care professionals, public health professionals, the public	Ad hoc	Regularly updated

NOTES: ACIP = Advisory Committee on Immunization Practices; COCA = Clinician Outreach and Communication Activity; MMWR = *Morbidity and Mortality Weekly Report*; PHE = public health emergency. CDC publications other than MMWRs are in Appendix E.
SOURCES: CDC, 2025a,b,c.

publicly available CDC vaccine safety communications, their purpose, primary audience, regular schedule, and total number produced during the PHE, if known. ACIP meetings, COCA calls, and *Morbidity and Mortality Weekly Reports* (MMWRs) regarding vaccine risk, harms, and safety monitoring increased significantly. ISO peer-reviewed publications other than MMWRs are discussed in Chapter 2, and a catalog is in Appendix E. During his presentation to the committee, Jernigan highlighted his partner newsletters as an important channel (over 152,000 subscribers received them from December 2020 to May 2023) (Jernigan, 2025), but these are not publicly available, and the committee was not provided with samples to review. Additionally, CDC shared vaccine safety information on social media platforms and received approximately 101 million views across Instagram, X, Facebook, and LinkedIn during the same time frame. Webpages were updated as additional information about vaccine safety and harms was identified from safety signals, such as thrombosis with thrombocytopenia syndrome (TTS), and social listening activities (Jernigan, 2025). CDC also used a variety of web sources, including social media platforms, online forums, blogs, and polls, to publish State of COVID-19 Vaccine Confidence Insights Reports.

ISO's communication remit has been scientific, not consumer facing—publishing safety analyses in peer-reviewed journals, presenting data to ACIP, and issuing MMWR summaries. CDC itself notes that ISO "regularly shares vaccine safety monitoring findings through presentations at scientific meetings and publication in peer-reviewed journals," while ACIP converts those data into vaccination policy guidance. After the U.S. COVID vaccines were authorized and recommended for use in December 2020, ISO staff responded to safety concerns raised by HCPs, public health officials, and the public (Miller et al., 2023). Inquiries were received primarily through CDC-INFO (a telephone and email system that responds to general questions for CDC) and CDC's National Immunization Program (an email service that responds to general questions about immunization); inquiries that require vaccine safety expertise are triaged to the ISO vaccine safety inquiry response program, staffed by nurses, physicians, epidemiologists, and other health scientists with expertise in vaccine safety (Miller et al., 2023). Between December 1, 2020, and August 31, 2022, ISO received 1,655 inquiries about COVID vaccine safety, with the most common about deaths after vaccination (160, 10 percent), myocarditis and related topics (153, 9 percent); pregnancy and reproductive health outcomes (123, 7 percent); understanding or interpreting data from the Vaccine Adverse Event Reporting System (VAERS) (111, 7 percent); and TTS and related questions about blood clotting (95, 6 percent) (Miller et al., 2023).

The COVID response was agencywide, established at the direction of the CDC director, and part of a larger multiagency incident command structure within the Department of Health and Human Services (HHS)

TABLE 3-2 CDC COVID-19 Vaccine Safety Task Force Teams

COVID-19 Vaccine Safety Team (VST)
• ISO staff deployed to this team • Relied on rotating deployers from across the agency • >200 deployers to the VST during the response • Typically, 6–8-week deployments • Spring 2022: Response activities transition to program (ISO)
COVID-19 Vaccine Communications Team
• Worked with COVID-19 VST on vaccine-related communications • Team size varying from 2 to 10 deployers   ○ Typically 4–8-week deployments • October 2020–Spring 2022: Deployment of health communication specialists within CDC • Summer 2021: Permanent FTE and DHQP contracted staff dedicated vaccine safety communications

NOTES: DHQP = Division of Healthcare Quality and Promotion; FTE = full-time employee; ISO = Immunization Safety Office; VST = Vaccine Safety Team. The Vaccine Task Force included new systems and activities, including V-safe, COVID-19 Vaccine Pregnancy Registry, follow-up of long-term effects of myocarditis, long-term care facility monitoring, and development of ACIP COVID-19 Vaccine Safety Technical Working Group (VaST) (Su, 2024).
SOURCE: Prepared by the committee and adapted from the presentation by Daniel Jernigan, 2025.

and overall federal government. CDC staff were deployed or temporarily assigned to assist with response efforts. Various task forces were formed as part of the scientific response section, including epidemiology and surveillance, modeling, and the Vaccine Task Force, which contained the COVID-19 Vaccine Safety Team (VST) and COVID-19 Vaccine Communications Team (established during summer 2020, Figure 3-2). ISO staff, in addition to CDC staff from NCIRD—and other parts of the agency based on their skills and knowledge—were deployed to the COVID-19 VST.

The vaccine safety communication products clearance process is similar during emergency and routine times, with a few key differences (Jernigan, 2025) (see Figure 3-3). During nonemergency periods (also referred to as "routine"), the level of clearance and need for cross-clearance within CDC depends on the product; ISO vaccine safety communications—focused on risk and harms—are often combined with vaccine use and recommendation communications from centers within CDC, such as NCIRD, in the context of risks versus benefits. During the PHE, the CDC joint information center was the central point of information coordination and emergency risk communication; its functions included centralizing and developing a strategy for response communications, staffing, engaging with clinician and nonclinician partners, response clearance, and research and evaluation (Jernigan, 2025). Jernigan explained that ISO's mandate is to identify and communicate

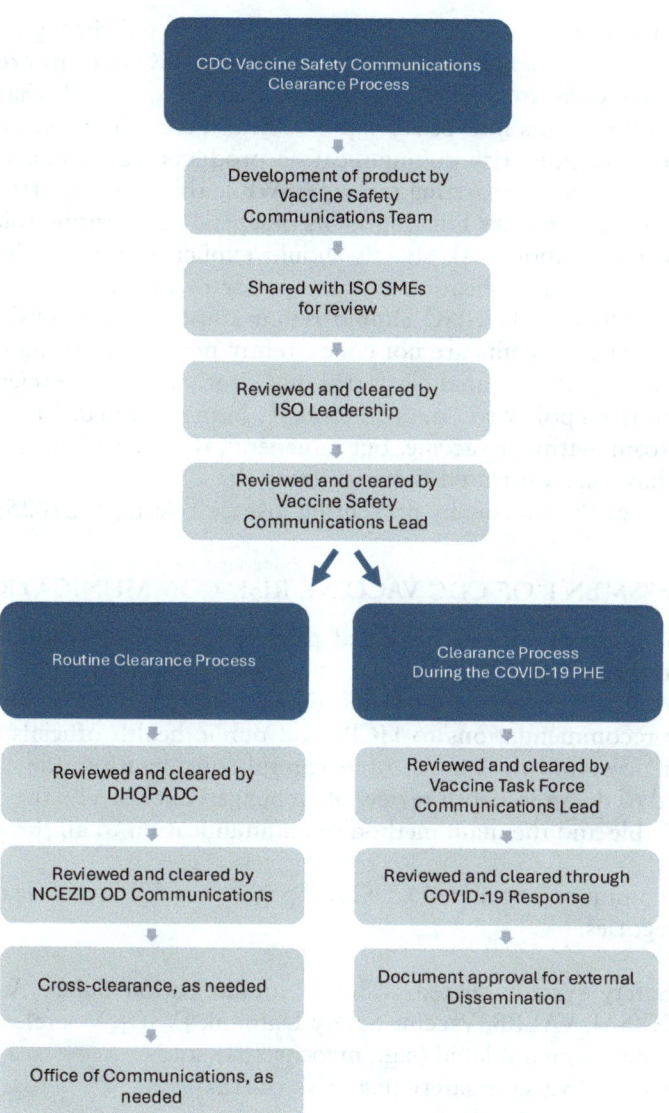

FIGURE 3-3 CDC vaccine safety communications routine clearance process vs. clearance process during the COVID public health emergency.
NOTE: ADC = Associate Director of Communications; DHQP = Division of Healthcare Quality and Promotion; ISO = Immunization Safety Office; NCEZID = National Center for Emerging and Zoonotic Infectious Diseases; OD = Office of the Director; SME = subject-matter expert.
SOURCE: Prepared by the committee and adapted from the presentation by Daniel Jernigan, 2025.

potential risks from vaccines—such as signals detected through its safety systems—without engaging in vaccine promotion. ISO aims to present this information clearly, in ways that help individuals understand what a signal means and how it fits into broader public health considerations. However, during the pandemic, risk communication products were frequently combined with benefit-emphasizing messages. While this framing may aid decision making, it also risks blurring ISO's independent scientific role. Future communications about risk signals should explicitly distinguish between ISO's role in risk identification and the policy or promotional messaging issued by CDC or HHS. ISO should retain authority to publish its findings—even when benefits are not concurrently presented—using standardized templates and dedicated platforms that clearly demarcate scientific risk assessment from policy recommendation. As Jernigan noted, "there is a risk of harm from getting a vaccine, but in general, these licensed or approved vaccines have demonstrated that risk from that vaccine is outweighed by the benefits of the vaccine by preventing disease" (Jernigan, 2025).

ASSESSMENT OF CDC VACCINE RISK COMMUNICATIONS

The Statement of Task specified that the committee would evaluate CDC external communications about its safety monitoring systems, the findings of COVID vaccine safety monitoring, and vaccination and clinical guidance recommendations to HCPs and public health officials ("technical" audiences) and the public. After careful consideration, the committee proceeded to do an in-depth review of webpages, exclusively; they are publicly available and the main method of communication to all three priority audiences.

The committee evaluated CDC webpages that fell into at least one of three categories:

- Safety system related (Clinical Immunization Safety Assessment [CISA], VAERS, Vaccine Safety Datalink [VSD], V-safe),
- Safety signal related (e.g., myocarditis), and
- General vaccine safety (e.g., risk of AEs).

As a result of its Moving Forward initiative, CDC launched Clean Slate, to "overhaul the CDC.gov website and streamline content by more than 60 percent so that people will be better able to find the information they're looking for to protect their health" (CDC, 2024a). Many webpages that were active during the PHE were archived; new webpages were created, though many of them contained content from the archived ones. The committee reviewed all webpages (archived or active) that were safety system related, about general vaccine safety, and regarding AEs and safety signals after receiving a COVID vaccine.

In 2015, the U.S. Web Design System was established from executive initiatives as a collaboration between the U.S. Digital Service and 18F[3] (Miller, 2025), a digital services agency within the General Services Administration (GSA, 2015). The goal is to provide a set of common visual and technical elements for federal websites, aiming to offer high-quality, consistent digital experiences. Due to this ongoing improvement initiative, the committee did not evaluate CDC webpages for any standards or elements under its purview.[4]

Additionally, the committee hosted a public listening session to gather stakeholder input on CDC's vaccine safety research and communications. During this 2-hour virtual session, preregistered attendees were given up to 3 minutes each to share their perspectives and recommendations (see Box 1-4 for a summary of salient points). It invited public comment on ways to improve CDC's research—both during PHEs and in routine vaccination contexts—and make information about vaccine safety and risks more accessible and understandable. Topics included criteria for evaluating potential harms, the timing and communication of emerging safety signals, and strategies to strengthen public confidence in vaccines.

In parallel, the committee contracted with an independent third party to conduct confidential key informant interviews. These interviews engaged a diverse group of stakeholders to obtain in-depth insights on CDC's current approaches and identify areas for improvement in vaccine safety monitoring and communication (see Appendix C).

Approach

The committee adapted its approach to webpage evaluation from specific guidelines for communicators described by Covello (2021): for creating clear technical information, delivering clear technical information, and enhancing the clarity of technical information. The following principles of effective communication were considered:

---

[3] On March 1, 2025, 18F was eliminated as part of a federal reorganization (Miller, 2025).

[4] As of September 26, 2024, federal website standards are available at standards.digital.gov. Federal agencies are required to comply with these standards per the 21st Century Integrated Digital Experience Act (IDEA) (2018), which made federal government website modernization a legal requirement. The standards are developed through a rigorous and iterative process involving federal agencies, the public, and other relevant groups. Each standard includes acceptance criteria that specify what elements must be present to be compliant. The status of each standard reflects its stage in the development process: research, draft, pending, or required (GSA, n.d.a,b).

- Avoids or appropriately uses technical or bureaucratic jargon, acronyms, and abbreviations;
- Uses culturally relevant, meaningful and linguistically appropriate language (words in the language they understand);
- Defines new or key terms so the target audience can understand them;
- Uses brief and clear sentences, particularly when defining new terms;
- Summarizes key information and is prominently placed;
- Provides focused message points;
- Provides complex information in tiers or layers of information that increase gradually in complexity; and
- Clearly communicates the science upon which the information is based.

The committee also assessed whether a webpage contained appropriate and meaningful visuals/graphics that enhance the text.

As mentioned, ISO's risk communication is often interwoven into broader vaccine safety messaging—including risk of harms in the context of benefits—and this was a common observation for the committee as it reviewed webpages that did not exclusively include information about risk and harms. As a result, the evaluation assesses risk communications regardless of authorship. However, webpages regarding ISO's vaccine safety systems—CISA, VAERS, VSD, and V-safe—are strictly within its purview and assumed authorship.

After its assessment, the committee found that its observations fell primarily into the guiding principles (discussed in Chapter 1) of relevance (communication activities meaningfully addressing the needs of health professionals, policy makers, and the public), credibility (the production and dissemination of scientifically sound information about vaccine risks), and independence (communications are free from undue internal or external influence).

Assumption of a Baseline Level of Technical Knowledge

The committee's assessment revealed that many vaccine safety webpages present information in a way that assumes readers have a certain level of technical background, though that assumption should not be applied universally. Technical audiences are not experts in communicating risk (Jones et al., 2025) and would benefit from using plain language with more accessible explanations of technical concepts regardless of audience. For example, a webpage that describes CDC's vaccine safety monitoring program (CDC, 2024b) does not clearly explain what vaccine safety monitoring is, and a page that describes how it works (CDC, 2024c) assumes knowledge of vaccine safety science.

Inconsistency and Discrepancy in Definitions

Key terms, such as "risk," "adverse events," "adverse events of special interest," "side effects," "complex safety questions," "safety signal," and "safety concern" are not defined at all, used inconsistently across content, or used in ways that could be misinterpreted without context. For example, "vaccine adverse event" is used differently across contexts, contributing to public confusion. In VAERS, it refers to any health problem occurring after vaccination, whether or not it is causally related. However, the name "Vaccine Adverse Event Reporting System" can imply to the public that all reported events are caused by vaccines. Public-facing materials should more clearly explain that VAERS accepts all reports to ensure early detection of rare issues—not because all events are vaccine related. Similarly, risk language used across CDC materials varied in specificity. Some risks (e.g., TTS ≈ 4 per million doses) were numerically defined, while others (e.g., myocarditis) were described qualitatively. Standardizing terminology and ensuring consistent risk quantification would improve clarity (CDC, 2025d). Moreover, safety monitoring during the pandemic was described as using established systems, but one of the extensively used systems (V-safe) was created during the PHE (CDC, 2024d).

Lack of Accessible Information

The committee found a lack of accessible information regarding the science and research methods behind the processes, systems, and conclusions related to potential vaccine-related harms. Some webpages provided appropriate safety information to technical audiences but could have included more substantive information that clearly explained the underlying science. Some cases had limited context or explanation for certain statements, such as "most intensive safety monitoring in U.S. history" (CDC, 2025e). This claim requires supporting evidence, particularly considering the public's resistance to blanket statements. The VSD webpage assumes the audience has familiarity with public health and analytic methods without necessarily explaining them (CDC, 2024e). Additionally, several webpages link to technical articles regarding vaccine safety on PubMed; this may lead some members of the public to disengage and may have restricted access if articles were behind a paywall.

Organization and Structure

The organization and structure of vaccine safety webpages presented difficulties in navigation functionality. A structural observation in the committee's assessment highlighted challenges in the design: Webpages did not clearly indicate whether the content was intended for a technical or lay audience.[5] This lack of clarity made navigation especially difficult, particularly when pages were linked to others that may have targeted different audiences. Numerous webpages also contain similar content, which can hinder users' ability to navigate effectively and recall key information.

Broader Context of Information About Potential Vaccine-Related Harmful Outcomes

As discussed in Chapter 1, ISO's function is to provide information to health professionals, policy makers, and the public regarding vaccine safety (see Box 1-3), focused on vaccine risks. As mentioned, the committee observed that vaccine safety information is often presented alongside the benefits to help contextualize potential risks and harms. As a result, some of the committee's observations are outside the purview of ISO but would aid CDC in providing effective communication about potential vaccine-related health outcomes to necessary audiences. Public health communication often relies on simplified messaging to promote clarity and action. However, this approach can obscure the nuance inherent in vaccine safety data, particularly during novel disease outbreaks where scientific understanding evolves rapidly. In such cases, changes in guidance should be seen as not institutional failure but rather a reflection of transparency, new evidence, and real-time learning. Communicating this iterative nature of science—while preserving public trust—is a persistent challenge for vaccine safety offices and communicators alike (Fischhoff et al., 2014, 2019; Han et al., 2021). To address this, ongoing communication research is necessary to understand how best to communicate vaccine safety information within this dynamic environment. Ultimately, attending to the areas outlined next can aid in building public trust while navigating the nuanced landscape of vaccine safety data.

---

[5] Before May 15, 2025, webpage content did not consistently indicate whether it was intended for a technical or lay audience. After this date, the committee started to observe the addition of clarifying labels, such as "For Everyone" or "For Healthcare Professionals," to indicate general audience orientation.

Tailored Information

Vaccine safety communication efforts are intentionally designed to effectively share evidence-based information, address concerns, and build trust (Jernigan, 2025). Collaborating with trusted messengers and key opinion leaders was a core strategy for effective public engagement during the pandemic. Jernigan (2025) explained that these messengers can be religious and/or community leaders and partners, individuals proficient in various languages who can ensure messages are received accurately and appropriately, and HCPs. The committee found very few webpages geared toward providing these trusted lay messengers with information that would equip them with the knowledge, skills, and tools necessary to communicate effectively about vaccine risks. This is especially true for historically underserved and underrepresented groups. While CDC emphasized the role of national messengers and partner organizations, state and local health departments were often better positioned to engage community leaders and respond in real time. State and local agencies actively pushed vaccine-related information through trusted local figures, including clergy, teachers, and neighborhood organizations. These efforts, rooted in community relationships, sometimes outpaced or compensated for delayed or generic federal communications. Future strategies should more clearly define and support the complementary roles of CDC and state agencies in messaging. Additionally, ensuring that webpages are tailored to not only a broader array of trusted messengers but also lay audiences would improve the effectiveness of evidence-based communication and enhance credibility.

Tailoring may take one of two forms: (a) risk information for a specific demographic and (b) messages that are culturally responsive to communities' specific concerns. Efforts to tailor information were hindered by incomplete demographic data. For example, race and ethnicity data were missing from more than half of the vaccine records reported to some states, limiting the ability to target communication strategies to disproportionately affected communities or evaluate equity in outreach (CDC, 2021a). Addressing these data gaps is essential for ensuring that vaccine safety communication is inclusive, equitable, and evidence based.

It was unclear to the committee exactly what efforts were taken to be culturally responsive. Moving forward, integrating community-engaged findings and feedback as part of the communications process will help ensure the relevance of vaccine safety information.

Communication with the Public

CDC emphasized the importance of understanding what the community is hearing or saying. Especially during the PHE, it used social listening, defined by Stewart and Arnold (2017) as "an active process of attending to, observing, interpreting, and responding to a variety of stimuli through mediated, electronic, and social channels" and published State of Vaccine Confidence Insights Reports to share what it observed with partners and the public. Information on CDC's Myths & Facts About COVID-19 Vaccines webpage may have also come from social listening, although it is not explicitly stated (CDC, 2024f). However, social listening is not necessarily bidirectional communication. The committee is particularly unclear about the processes to ensure the insights gained are incorporated into communication materials (and if ISO used any inquiries described by Miller et al. (2023) to create such materials, discussed earlier in the chapter).

Throughout the pandemic, social media platforms, visual dashboards, and scientific journals were used to disseminate vaccine safety findings. However, most communications remained one directional, lacking mechanisms for real-time, bidirectional engagement with the public. To meet evolving communication expectations, CDC and ISO should explore new formats—such as interactive explainers, Q&A forums, and multimedia summaries—to convey complex vaccine safety data. These tools should be accessible on mobile platforms and optimized for different audience types. Traditional methods, like the MMWR, remain indispensable for professional audiences, but they are poorly suited for public understanding without translation. Innovative formats should be used not to replace but to complement core scientific communications.

The process for public comment on ACIP recommendations is governed by federal requirements (Federal Advisory Committee Act and Office of Management and Budget directives) to ensure transparency and public participation in decision making (GSA, 2025). ACIP meetings must be announced in the Federal Register at least 15 calendar days in advance and include meeting dates and times, topics to be discussed, and instructions for the public to register for oral comment or submit written comments. The committee performed a high-level review of written public comments submitted through the Federal Register before the standing February 2021 (CDC, 2021b), June 2021 (CDC, 2021c,d), and October 2021 (CDC, 2021e) ACIP meetings.[6] Given the volume of comments related to vaccine risks and harms, the committee believes this may be a valuable avenue for ISO to explore—in not only gathering feedback from diverse audiences but also incorporating it into communication materials.

A critical but often underarticulated communication vulnerability lies in blurring ISO's mission—focused on vaccine risk surveillance—with broader immunization promotion efforts. When communications about

---

[6] These were the three scheduled meetings in 2021. The first COVID vaccine was authorized for emergency use on December 11, 2020.

ISO's findings are closely coupled with or filtered through policy advocacy or vaccine promotion, it may unintentionally undermine the perceived independence of ISO's safety monitoring role, particularly among individuals already predisposed to skepticism (Larson et al., 2014; Quinn et al., 2019). This dynamic can erode public trust in vaccine safety assessments, even when the underlying science is rigorous and the intent transparent. To safeguard trust and reinforce ISO's credibility, it ought to be equipped with independent communication channels specifically dedicated to sharing its safety surveillance processes, evaluation criteria, and findings—separate from CDC's promotional or policy-facing content. Clearly delineated, plain-language communications about what ISO does and how it does it would not only improve transparency but also help insulate its work from misperceptions of bias or agenda alignment.

CONCLUSION

The COVID PHE compelled CDC's ISO to release vaccine risk information at a speed and scale never before required. ISO and its communication partners produced a vast body of technical content—on safety signals, monitoring systems, and analytic methods—that clinicians and health officials found indispensable for day-to-day decision making. Yet the committee observed that this content was usually embedded in broader CDC messaging and cleared through processes that emphasized vaccine uptake goals, blurring ISO's independent scientific voice and, at times, limiting public visibility into how safety findings were generated and released. The committee used the five guiding principles to frame its analysis and recommendations, and its conclusion on ISO's communication activities is organized according to those same principles.

Relevance: ISO's webpages often assume professional familiarity with epidemiologic concepts, provide few cues about their intended audience, and nest critical definitions several clicks deep. Navigation is further hampered by multiple pages that repeat similar content or mix lay and technical language. To make future outputs meaningfully useful, ISO ought to segment products by audience, layer detail, and ensure that trusted messengers—especially those serving underserved communities—can quickly locate plain-language explanations that match what they hear through social listening and public comment channels.

Credibility: The underlying science is sound, but inconsistent terminology ("adverse event," "safety signal," "risk") and nonstandardized risk metrics impede interpretation and increase the danger of misunderstanding, incorrect interpretation, and misuse of data. Publishing study protocols, explicitly defining key terms, and adopting a single risk-reporting template across all AEs would let external reviewers verify methods and enhance public trust.

Data stewardship: ISO relies on individuals and health care systems that contribute sensitive data to VAERS, VSD, V-safe, and CISA. The committee saw little public-facing material that explains how privacy is safeguarded or how outside researchers can request controlled access to deidentified data—an omission that may undercut the social license to operate these systems. Making stewardship practices and data-sharing pathways more transparent would honor participants and widen the scientific lens on vaccine safety.

Continuous improvement and innovation: ISO rapidly adopted social media "listening," new visual templates, and the U.S. Web Design System during the pandemic, demonstrating an ability to modernize. Embedding usability metrics, readability goals, and routine user testing and input into the forthcoming strategic plan will institutionalize that agility, ensuring that communications evolve alongside novel vaccine platforms, new data streams, an evolving information environment, and emerging best practices in risk messaging.

Independence: The most consistent theme in public comments and key informant interviews was the erosion of trust that occurs when safety findings appear filtered through benefit-promotion lenses. ISO content is still cross-cleared with offices whose mission is to increase vaccine uptake, and webpages frequently couple risk estimates with exhortations to vaccinate. To protect scientific integrity, CDC ought to firewall ISO communications from policy and promotional channels, give ISO scientists final authority to post risk analyses—even when benefits are not simultaneously discussed—and brand those postings on a distinct ISO platform. Doing so will clarify roles, shorten time to publication, and reassure skeptical audiences that safety evidence is reported fully and without spin. To advance transparency and structural clarity, ISO's communications should be operationally insulated from benefit–risk determinations and promotional content. During the pandemic, publication delays sometimes arose due to clearance processes that required cross-office approvals. Streamlining ISO's ability to independently publish risk findings—backed by transparent data and standardized protocols—would bolster public trust and speed the translation of emerging signals into policy deliberation.

Despite the strength and coordination of the underlying vaccine safety infrastructure, the committee finds that communication about how the system functioned—and safety findings were evaluated and disseminated—was insufficiently transparent. Even among internal stakeholders (Edwards et al., 2025), it was not always clear how risk assessments were communicated to the public or which channels were used to share evolving findings. For the general public, the structure and rigor of the vaccine safety monitoring, evaluation, and communication were rarely explained coherently and accessibly. This lack of transparency weakened confidence in the system and hindered appreciation of the extensive behind-the-scenes efforts to monitor and ensure vaccine safety. Greater clarity about the surveillance systems, evaluation processes, and decision-making criteria—particularly during emergencies—should be a standing priority.

Finally, the committee acknowledges the need for coherent and coordinated communication in a landscape that includes multiple surveillance systems, external collaborators, and a rapid pace of discovery. During the COVID response, ISO and its partners operated under intense scrutiny and pressure to deliver timely findings. In this context, the need to align messages across agencies and programs sometimes conflicted with the expectations of scientific independence held by non-government investigators. The federal clearance process, while intended to promote message consistency, occasionally led to concerns about the suppression or delay of legitimate scientific findings. Balancing the imperative for communication discipline with the values of transparency and investigator autonomy will be critical for public trust. Establishing clear, publicly available criteria for when and how findings are communicated—especially for research conducted in collaboration with academic or non-federal institutions—can help strike this balance.

ISO's ability to detect and explain vaccine risks is crucial for national and global immunization programs. Strengthening relevance through audience-specific content, enhancing credibility with standardized methods, demonstrating respect for data contributors, institutionalizing continuous improvement, and, critically, asserting operational independence will make ISO the definitive, trusted voice on vaccine risk science—both in routine times and during the next public health crisis.

REFERENCES

Brewer, N. T., G. B. Chapman, A. J. Rothman, J. Leask, and A. Kempe. 2017. Increasing vaccination: Putting psychological science into action. *Psychological Science in the Public Interest* 18(3):149–207. https://doi.org/10.1177/1529100618760521.

CDC (Centers for Disease Control and Prevention). 2021a. *Demographic characteristics of persons vaccinated during the first month of the COVID-19 vaccination program—United States, December 14, 2020–January 14, 2021.* https://www.cdc.gov/mmwr/volumes/70/wr/mm7005e1.htm (accessed August 6, 2025).

CDC. 2021b. *Advisory Committee on Immunization Practices.* Washington, DC: Centers for Disease Control and Prevention. https://www.federalregister.gov/documents/2021/01/27/2021-01737/advisory-committee-on-immunization-practices-acip (accessed August 26, 2025).

CDC. 2021c. *Advisory Committee on Immunization Practices (ACIP) June 23–24 2021.* https://www.regulations.gov/document/CDC-2021-0034-0001 (accessed June 16, 2025).

CDC. 2021d. *Advisory Committee on Immunization Practices (ACIP); Amended Notice of Meeting.* https://www.federalregister.gov/documents/2021/07/02/2021-14203/advisory-committee-on-immunization-practices-acip-amended-notice-of-meeting (accessed June 16, 2025).

CDC. 2021e. *Advisory Committee on Immunization Practices (ACIP); Amended Notice of Meeting.* https://www.federalregister.gov/documents/2021/11/08/2021-24320/advisory-committee-on-immunization-practices-acip-amended-notice-of-meeting (accessed September 10, 2025).
CDC. 2024a. *CDC moving forward.* https://www.cdc.gov/about/cdc-moving-forward.html (accessed April 16, 2025).
CDC. 2024b. *About CDC's Vaccine Safety Monitoring Program.* https://www.cdc.gov/vaccine-safety-systems/about/cdc-monitoring-program.html (accessed April 24, 2025).
CDC. 2024c. *How vaccine safety monitoring works.* https://www.cdc.gov/vaccine-safety-systems/about/monitoring.html (accessed April 24, 2025).
CDC. 2024d. About V-safe. https://www.cdc.gov/vaccine-safety-systems/v-safe/index.html (accessed September 10, 2025).
CDC. 2024e. Vaccine Safety Datalink (VSD). https://www.cdc.gov/vaccine-safety-systems/vsd/ (accessed August, 7, 2025).
CDC. 2024f. *Myths & facts about COVID-19 vaccines.* https://www.cdc.gov/covid/vaccines/myths-facts.html (accessed April 24, 2025).
CDC. 2025a. *COCA calls.* https://www.cdc.gov/coca/hcp/trainings/index.html (accessed April 16, 2025).
CDC. 2025b. *About the Morbidity and Mortality Weekly Report (MMWR) series.* https://www.cdc.gov/mmwr/about.html (accessed August 6, 2025).
CDC. 2025c. *ACIP meeting information.* https://www.cdc.gov/acip/meetings/index.html (accessed August 8, 2025).
CDC. 2025d. Coronavirus disease 2019 (COVID-19) vaccine safety. https://www.cdc.gov/vaccine-safety/vaccines/covid-19.html (accessed September 10, 2025).
CDC. 2025e. COVID-19 vaccine safety reporting systems. https://www.cdc.gov/vaccine-safety-systems/monitoring/covid-19.html (accessed September 10, 2025).
Covello, V. T. 2021. *Communicating in risk, crisis, and high stress situations: Evidence-based strategies and practice.* Piscataway, NJ: John Wiley & Sons.
Dolman, A. J., T. Fraser, C. Panagopoulos, D. P. Aldrich, and D. Kim. 2023. Opposing views: Associations of political polarization, political party affiliation, and social trust with COVID-19 vaccination intent and receipt. *Journal of Public Health* 45(1):36–39. https://doi.org/10.1093/pubmed/fdab401.
Dubé, E., and N. E. MacDonald. 2017. Vaccination resilience: Building and sustaining confidence in and demand for vaccination. *Vaccine* 35(32):3907–3909. https://doi.org/10.1016/j.vaccine.2017.06.015.
Dudley, M. Z., B. Schwartz, J. Brewer, L. Kan, R. Bernier, J. E. Gerber, H. B. Ni, T. M. Proveaux, R. N. Rimal, and D. A. Salmon. 2022. COVID-19 vaccination status, attitudes, and values among U.S. adults in September 2021. *Journal of Clinical Medicine* 11(13):3734. https://doi.org/10.3390/jcm11133734.
Edwards, J., N. Osuoha, J. Maizel, R. Neenan, N. Page, P. Resichmann, and B. Slotman. 2025. *Key informant interviews findings report.* Rockville, MD: Westat.
Eller, N. M., N. B. Henrikson, and D. J. Opel. 2019. Vaccine information sources and parental trust in their child's health care provider. *Health Education & Behavior* 46(3):445–453. https://doi.org/10.1177/1090198118819716.
Fischhoff, B. 2019. Evaluating science communication. *Proceedings of the National Academy of Sciences* 116(16):7670–7675. https://doi.org/10.1073/pnas.1805863115.
Fischhoff, B., and A. L. Davis. 2014. Communicating scientific uncertainty. *Proceedings of the National Academy of Sciences* 111(supplement_4):13664–13667. https://doi.org/110.1073/pnas.1317504111.
Fraser, M. 2023. ASTHO response to Senate help request for information on CDC reform October 20, 2023.

French, J., S. Deshpande, W. Evans, and R. Obregon. 2020. Key guidelines in developing a pre-emptive COVID-19 vaccination uptake promotion strategy. *International Journal of Environmental Research and Public Health* 17(16):5893. https://doi.org/10.3390/ijerph17165893.

GSA (General Services. Administration). n.d.a. *Federal website standards: About.* https://standards.digital.gov/about/ (accessed April 12, 2025).

GSA. n.d.b. *Federal website standards: Standards.* https://standards.digital.gov/standards/ (accessed April 12, 2025).

GSA. 2015. *Introducing the U.S. Web Design Standards.* https://18f.gsa.gov/2015/09/28/web-design-standards/ (archived on February 27, 2025, using the Wayback Machine: https://web.archive.org/web/20250227225756/).

GSA. 2025. *Federal advisory committee act (FACA) management overview.* https://www.gsa.gov/policy-regulations/policy/federal-advisory-committee-management (accessed April 24, 2025).

Hammershaimb, E. A., J. D. Campbell, and S. T. O'Leary. 2022. Coronavirus disease-2019 vaccine hesitancy. *Pediatric Clinics of North America* 70(2):243. https://doi.org/10.1016/j.pcl.2022.12.001.

Han, P. K., E. Scharnetzki, A. M. Scherer, A. Thorpe, C. Lary, L. B. Waterston, A. Fagerlin, and N. F. Dieckmann. 2021. Communicating scientific uncertainty about the COVID-19 pandemic: Online experimental study of an uncertainty-normalizing strategy. *Journal of Medical Internet Research* 23(4):e2783210.2196/27832.

Jernigan, D. 2025. CDC COVID-19 vaccine safety risk communications. Presentation to the Committee to Review the Centers for Disease Control and Prevention's COVID-19 Vaccine Safety Research and Communications, Washington, DC, January 10, 2025.

Jones, M., S. Ratzan, and R. Tuckson. 2025. Challenges and opportunities for research and communication about vaccine safety. Washington, DC, February 25.

Juanchich, M., C. M. Oakley, H. Sayer, D. L. Holford, W. Bruine de Bruin, C. Booker, T. Chadborn, G. Vallee-Tourangeau, R. M. Wood, and M. Sirota. 2024. Vaccination invitations sent by warm and competent medical professionals disclosing risks and benefits increase trust and booking intention and reduce inequalities between ethnic groups. *Health Psychology.*

Larson, H. J., C. Jarrett, E. Eckersberger, D. M. Smith, and P. Paterson. 2014. Understanding vaccine hesitancy around vaccines and vaccination from a global perspective: A systematic review of published literature, 2007–2012. *Vaccine* 32(19):2150–2159. https://doi.org/10.1016/j.vaccine.2014.01.081.

Miller, E. R., P. L. Moro, T. T. Shimabukuro, G. Carlock, S. N. Davis, E. M. Freeborn, A. L. Roberts, J. Gee, A. W. Taylor, R. Gallego, T. Suragh, and J. R. Su. 2023. COVID-19 vaccine safety inquiries to the Centers for Disease Control and Prevention Immunization Safety Office. *Vaccine* 41(27):3960–3963. https://doi.org/10.1016/j.vaccine.2023.05.054.

Miller, J. 2025. *After rocky history, GSA shuts down 18F office.* https://federalnewsnetwork.com/reorganization/2025/03/after-rocky-history-gsa-shuts-down-18f-office/ (accessed April 22, 2025).

Nowak, G. J., B. G. Gellin, N. E. MacDonald, and R. Butler. 2015. Addressing vaccine hesitancy: The potential value of commercial and social marketing principles and practices. *Vaccine* 33(34):4204–4211. https://doi.org/10.1016/j.vaccine.2015.04.039.

Nowak, G. J., A. K. Shen, and J. L. Schwartz. 2017. Using campaigns to improve perceptions of the value of adult vaccination in the United States: Health communication considerations and insights. *Vaccine* 35(42):5543–5550.

Quinn, S. C., A. M. Jamison, J. An, G. R. Hancock, and V. S. Freimuth. 2019. Measuring vaccine hesitancy, confidence, trust and flu vaccine uptake: Results of a national survey of White and African American adults. *Vaccine* 37(9):1168–1173. https://doi.org/10.1016/j.vaccine.2019.01.033.

Reyna, V. F., W. L. Nelson, P. K. Han, and N. F. Dieckmann. 2009. How numeracy influences risk comprehension and medical decision making. *Psychological Bulletin* 135(6):943.

Sarathchandra, D., and J. Johnson-Leung. 2024. How political ideology and media shaped vaccination intention in the early stages of the COVID-19 pandemic in the United States. *COVID* 4(5):658–671. https://doi.org/10.3390/covid4050045.

Stewart, M. C., and C. L. Arnold. 2017. Defining social listening: Recognizing an emerging dimension of listening. *International Journal of Listening* 32(2):85–100 https://doi.org/10.1080/10904018.2017.1330656.

Su, J. R. 2024. U.S. Centers for Disease Control and Prevention COVID-19 vaccine safety monitoring from December 2020—May 2023. Presentation to the Committee to Review the Centers for Disease Control and Prevention's COVID-19 Vaccine Safety Research and Communications, Washington, DC, June 24, 2024.

Warren, A. M., M. M. Bennett, B. da Graca, A. C. Waddimba, R. L. Gottlieb, M. E. Douglas, and M. B. Powers. 2023. Intentions to receive COVID-19 vaccines in the United States: Sociodemographic factors and personal experiences with COVID-19. *Health Psychology* 42(8):531.

Zipkin, D. A., C. A. Umscheid, N. L. Keating, E. Allen, K. Aung, R. Beyth, S. Kaatz, D. M. Mann, J. B. Sussman, and D. Korenstein. 2014. Evidence-based risk communication: A systematic review. *Annals of Internal Medicine* 161(4):270–280. https://doi.org/10.7326/M14-0295.

4

Conclusions and Recommendations

The committee was charged to evaluate the activities of the Immunization Safety Office (ISO) during the COVID public health emergency (PHE) and provide recommendations for the future (see the Statement of Task in Box 1-1). Chapter 2 provides the review of the vaccine risk monitoring and evaluation work and Chapter 3 the communications activities. As described in Chapter 1, vaccine safety experts from ISO were detailed to the Vaccine Task Force at the Centers for Disease Control and Prevention (CDC) during the PHE. For convenience, this report refers to these staff, the systems they used, and the analytic approaches as "ISO," regardless of their organizational placement and reporting relationship at the time. Furthermore, the committee uses the phrase "vaccine risks" to indicate undesired, serious health outcomes. The use of "safety" indicates to some a complete lack of any negative outcomes and to some a balance between risks and benefits. ISO's primary role is to conduct ongoing surveillance and monitoring of vaccine safety, though it may also support hypothesis-driven research when needed to inform evaluation. Thus, the committee describes ISO's function as vaccine risk monitoring and evaluation.[1]

The committee does not want its focus on the risks of vaccines to detract from the overwhelming evidence of their benefits. One way to

---

[1] During the committee's deliberations, major changes were announced in the structure of CDC and its parent Department of Health and Human Services. To avoid possible confusion, the committee refers to ISO when describing the activities undertaken by that office before these reorganizations but to a federal vaccine risk monitoring and evaluation office for time periods after the start of those reorganizations.

increase use of vaccines when indicated, and therefore their benefits, is to increase understanding of and confidence in the studies of vaccine risks conducted by the federal government. The committee believes that ISO merits the nation's trust and serves as a reliable and unbiased source of monitoring, evaluation, and communication about vaccine risks. It offers recommendations to enhance ISO's capabilities.

As described briefly in Chapter 1, the committee identified five principles that ground its recommendations. A robust vaccine risk monitoring and evaluation office that merits the nation's trust needs to be relevant, seen as highly credible, trusted with data, committed to continuous improvement and innovation, and scientifically independent. These will be described in more detail in a subsequent section.

The committee offers three conclusions about the functioning of ISO, focusing on evidence about its activities during the PHE. The committee then offers five recommendations, framed around the aforementioned principles. The committee ends this chapter and report with overarching thoughts on the value of the office and its work.

CONCLUSIONS

Conclusion 4-1: ISO has played an important role performing and communicating about rigorous vaccine risk monitoring and evaluation.

Conclusion 4-2: In response to the COVID public health emergency declaration, ISO staff and systems produced and communicated an impressive quantity of timely, important, and high-quality monitoring, evaluation, and communication about COVID vaccine risks.

Conclusion 4-3: Trust in ISO as a credible source of vaccine risk information is affected by the intersection and interaction with CDC and other governmental efforts to foster vaccination. ISO currently lacks the organizational independence and resources to directly disseminate its information to health professionals, policy makers, and the public.

As documented in Chapter 2, ISO studies the risks of vaccines using standard pharmacoepidemiology, surveillance, and clinical research methods. The multiple systems for monitoring and evaluation are complementary, and the additional systems created during the PHE, such as V-safe, resulted in stronger monitoring and evaluation. Combined with vaccine safety evaluations as required by the Food and Drug Administration and the work of other federal agencies, such as the Veterans Health Administration and Centers for Medicare & Medicaid Services, and with regular communications and collaboration with international vaccine safety researchers, ISO is central to generating new knowledge about vaccine risks.

During the PHE, ISO conducted a large amount of timely and rigorous monitoring and evaluation (see Appendix E). As shown in the case studies in Appendix D, it made frequent public presentations of the findings as they emerged, helping health professionals, policy makers, and the public understand the effects of these vaccines in real time.

However, as the committee heard from public comments (see Box 1-5) and has been documented in studies of vaccine hesitancy, ISO research is viewed skeptically by some because of the intermingling of information about vaccine risks and benefits. Clearance of ISO risk publications currently involves those in CDC responsible for studying vaccine benefits and fostering immunization. Technical content was not solely reviewed by the risk experts (see Appendix C). Additionally, during the PHE, understandably, communications were cleared at multiple levels (Jernigan, 2025).

RECOMMENDATIONS

The committee identified a set of principles well established over decades that have influenced the functioning of a variety of federal statistical agencies and offices, including an office long housed at CDC, the National Center for Health Statistics (CDC, 2024; NASEM, 2025). The mutually reinforcing, co-equal principles articulated in this series of reports by the National Academies have been incorporated in federal directives and stood the test of time as a goal post for offices entrusted with citizens' data in service to the nation (NASEM, 2025).

The committee found the similarities in the functioning of federal statistical agencies to ISO compelling and, with a few changes in vocabulary to fit its specific task, uses those principles to frame recommendations for a robust vaccine risk monitoring and evaluation system that merits the nation's trust. It offers one recommendation related to each of the five principles and includes recommended implementation steps to guide future activities. Details about the implementation reside with the administration.

Relevance

Vaccine risk monitoring, evaluation, and communications activities meaningfully address the needs of health professionals, policy makers,[2] and the public.

---

[2] The committee intends policy makers to include federal, state, and local public health agencies.

> **BOX 4-1**
> **Principles of a Robust Vaccine Risk Monitoring and Evaluation System That Merits the Nation's Trust**
>
> Relevance: Vaccine risk monitoring, evaluation, and communications activities meaningfully address the needs of health professionals, policy makers, and the public.
>
> Credibility: Health professionals, policy makers, and the public can rely on scientifically sound information and data analysis about vaccine risks.
>
> Data stewardship: Vaccine risk monitoring, evaluation, and communication activities are conducted with respect for the individuals whose data are used by protecting their privacy, using the data properly to address important questions about vaccine risks, and sharing the results.
>
> Continuous improvement and innovation: Regular evaluation of vaccine risk monitoring, evaluation, and communication practices lead to adopting new methodologies and technologies with the capacity to address emerging questions about vaccine risks.
>
> Independence: Vaccine risk monitoring, evaluation, and communication are free from undue internal or external influence.

Recommendation 1: A robust vaccine risk monitoring and evaluation office should develop and make public a strategic plan that encompasses input from health professionals, policy makers, and the public to ensure that the plan is scientifically sound, meets the needs and expectations of those who use the information, and articulates the office's role in monitoring, evaluating, and communicating vaccine risks.

Implementation steps:

1. Include a clear mission statement.
2. Establish a board of scientific counselors.
3. Develop a scientific agenda.
4. Develop mechanisms for bidirectional communication with health professionals and the public.
5. Outline action steps that will be taken in a public health emergency.

The committee anchors its recommendation in a strategic plan and the processes established to develop it to ensure the work of the vaccine risk monitoring and evaluation office is relevant to health professionals, policy makers, and the public and that its mission is restricted to vaccine risk monitoring and evaluation and not promoting vaccine use. The office needs a simple, recognizable identity focused exclusively on vaccine risk monitoring and assessment. It can start by developing a mission statement, which the committee was unable to locate for ISO. A concise articulation of its focus on monitoring and evaluating the risks of vaccines could increase understanding of its work.

Any robust strategic plan is developed, reviewed, and revised on a regular basis and includes metrics for evaluation, timelines, and deadlines. It ought to include disclosure of the office's resources, such as staffing and research contracts. Transparency about the sources of funding for its resources is paramount in helping demonstrate the relevance of the office's work.

A key element of the plan is a scientific agenda. The committee is aware of an ISO research agenda published in 2011, developed in response to a recommendation by the Institute of Medicine (CDC, 2011; IOM, 2005) but none since. Outlining scientific priorities and reporting on progress is important for transparency and accountability. Soliciting input into the scientific agenda from health professionals and the public helps ensure it broadly represents the needs and interests of a range of interests. The input can take many forms—website, open comment sessions, and scientific workshops, for example. Articulating the strategy for decision making about what signals to pursue could assure health professionals, policy makers, and the public that issues of salience to them are not being ignored.

A board of scientific counselors can play an integral role in assuring credibility of the vaccine risk monitoring and evaluation office. The board would provide a locus for developing and reviewing the strategic plan, including the scientific agenda, serve as the conduit for communications with health professionals and the public, and support accountability. It would advise on the science and processes of vaccine risk monitoring, communications, and the independence of both of those functions, including that its products stay clear of policy and advocacy. The expertise of the board members ought to include, for example, an established track record in vaccinology, immunology, risk communication, vaccine safety, pharmacoepidemiology, and informatics. The office also should consider the merits of having a consumer or member of the public on the board. The head of the vaccine risk monitoring and evaluation office should have comparably deep and relevant expertise, in addition to skills as a communicator. Other roles for the board are articulated in subsequent sections.

Because vaccine risk monitoring and evaluation will follow compressed timelines and have unique scientific priorities during PHEs, the strategic plan ought to clearly indicate action steps to be taken to address the PHE and resource allocation, especially regarding personnel, and work that will be modified to address the emergency and maintain the routine work of the vaccine risk monitoring and evaluation office. Communications with health professionals and agencies at the state and local level is particularly important during an emergency.

Credibility

Health professionals, policy makers, and the public can rely on scientifically sound information and data analysis about vaccine risks.

Recommendation 2: A robust vaccine risk monitoring and evaluation office should be transparent and comprehensive in conducting and communicating its work in ways that are useful to health professionals, policy makers, and the public.

Implementation steps:

1. Focus on vaccine risk monitoring and evaluation, avoiding vaccine policymaking and promotion.
2. Develop a portfolio of publicly available information to explain systems and methodologic approaches, including data sources and system strengths and limitations, and priorities.
3. Ensure public availability of monitoring and evaluation protocols, including changes made during the data collection and analysis process and a justification for those changes.
4. Develop, disseminate, and evaluate accessible and easily understood plain language summaries of vaccine risk results.
5. Standardize risk reporting across communications and by risk groups, where available.

The work of a federal vaccine risk monitoring and evaluation office needs to be credible if the public is to trust it to assist in personal decision making. The committee heard during public comment period that some people mistrust the information from ISO because its parent agency, CDC, also promotes vaccines (see Box 1-5), a long-standing issue (CDC, 2004, 2006). As described in Chapter 3, CDC communications about vaccine risks usually include information about benefits, to portray the full picture of the effects. However, the committee thinks having a web presence for the work of the vaccine risk monitoring and evaluation office that clearly identifies the risk information distinct from vaccine advocacy or use recommendations could help some members of the public increase their trust in it. It could include links to CDC sites with use recommendations, effectiveness information, and general vaccine advocacy. The risk monitoring and evaluation experts ought to be consulted for technical accuracy, but other offices in CDC or HHS can use the risk information in policy determinations and communications

Two things that could help the public and health professionals trust information from this office are transparency and comprehensiveness. The public and those who promote and administer vaccines need to be able to understand the work of the office and trust what they see, knowing they are seeing the complete work. To facilitate public understanding of the work, the office ought to develop a suite of public-facing products, such as ones that explain the monitoring and evaluation systems used, including their strengths and limitations. The office should develop a process for explaining its decision making around studying risks of salience to the public. The board of scientific counselors can oversee this and provide advice.

An additional step toward transparency is to make the analysis protocols available (ISPE, 2015). The committee notes that some protocols from the Vaccine Safety Datalink (VSD) were made available during the PHE (CDC, 2023), but it has not been standard practice. Publishing research protocols is an integral part of clinical trials (NIH, 2025) and strongly recommended by pharmacoepidemiology experts (ISPE, 2025); the federal vaccine risk monitoring and evaluation office ought to adopt it as standard practice.

Because many people interested in vaccine risk evaluation do not have in-depth knowledge of epidemiology and statistics, this office ought to publish plain language summaries of every research publication and, where of broad national and public interest, unpublished findings that are made public, such as in public presentations. Additionally, where possible, to facilitate the public's understanding, the office ought to adopt standardized risk reporting, including relevant subgroup analyses where available.

Data Stewardship

Vaccine risk monitoring, evaluation, and communication activities are conducted with respect for the individuals whose data are used by protecting their privacy, using their data properly to address important questions about vaccine risks, and sharing the results.

Recommendation 3: A robust vaccine risk monitoring and evaluation office should be a good steward in the monitoring and evaluation processes by protecting the privacy of individuals and honoring their participation.

Implementation steps:

1. Protect personally identifiable information using appropriate standards.
2. Solicit input from researchers and the public about key elements of the research agenda.
3. Explore ways to make the data used in vaccine risk monitoring and evaluation more transparent and, where feasible and appropriate, available to external researchers.

Federal agencies have an obligation to be good stewards of the citizen information used for research and policymaking. Vaccine risk research depends on participation by a wide variety of individuals and their trust that their protected personal information is kept confidential. Private medical information and contact information are important to collect for research but ought not be made public. Members of the public whose information is included in systems such as the Vaccine Adverse Event Reporting System or VSD deserve to know that their data are secure.

Honoring their participation means that the public knows that they participate for a good reason—that the monitoring and evaluation questions being asked are important, addressed with appropriate scientific expertise, and broadly reflect the interests of the scientific community, health professionals, the public, and policy makers. The public input components of the research agenda and strategic plan for this office outlined in Recommendation 1 can help assure this. The monitoring and evaluation office contributes as much as possible with its given resources to understanding the risks of vaccines, but it is not, cannot, and should not be the only entity researching vaccine risks. The validity of the scientific process and the confidence in the results could be bolstered if, under appropriate circumstances, data collected and used by the office were available to outside researchers. VAERS data are available for free by download (VAERS, n.d.), and some limited VSD data had been available to outside researchers (CDC, n.d.). The board of scientific counselors envisioned in Recommendation 1 could provide the guidance and oversight of efforts to review and revise, if necessary, public access programs.

Continuous Improvement and Innovation

Regular evaluation of vaccine risk monitoring, evaluation, and communication practices leads to adopting new methodologies and technologies with the capacity to address emerging questions about vaccine risks.

Recommendation 4: A robust vaccine risk monitoring and evaluation office should integrate continuous quality improvements into its strategic plan to strengthen its activities.

Implementation steps:

1. Develop metrics for evaluation in conjunction with strategic plan and advisors.
2. Maintain current data monitoring and evaluation systems and activities while incorporating advances in informatics, vaccinology, and epidemiological and statistical methods.
3. Use communication research, including in risk communication, to inform and assess communications.

A well-functioning risk monitoring and evaluation office continuously improves and innovates. As with the first recommendation, metrics for evaluation ought to be developed that address innovation. The committee concluded that ISO has been important in performing and communicating about vaccine risk monitoring and evaluation and that during the PHE, its staff and the systems they used performed extremely well. Existing monitoring and evaluation systems ought to be continued and even enhanced and expanded as new information and new technologies become available. Implementing this and other recommendations will require resources, but the committee did not determine a specific level.

The board of scientific counselors described could oversee efforts by the office to incorporate advances in vaccinology, epidemiology and statistics, and informatics. Other federal partners can also provide input and collaborations, which are vital to scientifically robust monitoring and evaluation office. Additionally, as discussed in Chapter 3, the robust field of research on public health communication and risk communication could be leveraged to improve communication about vaccine risk monitoring and evaluation efforts by not only shaping communications but also evaluating them. It is important to assess how the messages are received by the intended audiences, particularly for helping the public understand uncertainty around emerging risks.

Independence

Vaccine risk monitoring, evaluation, and communication are free from undue internal or external influence.

Recommendation 5: The Centers for Disease Control and Prevention (CDC) should protect the scientific independence of its vaccine risk monitoring office and provide the administrative support and financial resources to conduct these activities.

Implementation steps:

1. Keep the vaccine risk monitoring and evaluation office organizationally and administratively separated from units in CDC that carry out administrative or policymaking activities, such as promoting vaccination.
2. Increase awareness of the vaccine risk monitoring and evaluation work by clearly distinguishing risk information from vaccine policy content and that intended to increase immunization.
3. Permit and encourage prompt publication of risk data.

Because the committee believes that vaccines have been demonstrated to provide enormous benefit to individuals and populations over the last century, it focuses on the scientific independence of risk monitoring and evaluation as a way to assure individuals and health professionals that the results are free from internal and external influence. The committee bases this not on evidence that the results have been tainted by association with vaccine promotion but because of the persistent perception that this is true (CDC, 2004, 2006). Unlike the preceding recommendations, this recommendation is directed to CDC; the risk monitoring and evaluation office cannot assure its own independence.

During its public comment session, the committee heard, as has been true for decades, that some fear the safety of vaccines because of the perception that risk research and communications are often inextricably linked to and biased by the CDC to increase vaccination (CDC, 2004) (see Box 1-5). While clinical use recommendations for vaccines, as with drugs, include considerations of benefits and risks and are clearly in the purview of the National Center for Immunization and Respiratory Diseases, ACIP, and other governmental offices, the risk information ought to be generated and communicated independently of efforts to increase immunization if it is to be trusted by those who do not currently. The committee notes, as described in Chapter 1, that annual funding for ISO has come from not only its parent center, but also NCIRD.[3]

---

[3] Personal communication, J. Gee, Centers for Disease Control and Prevention, August 5, 2025.

That office ought to remain, as ISO is, organizationally and administratively separated from those parts of the department that study vaccine benefits and work to increase vaccinations. The committee is aware of suggestions for alternative placements (Salmon et al., 2004) but did not evaluate these options, as that is outside of its remit. The office should have a web presence that is distinct from vaccine promotion efforts, clearly identifying the office from which the monitoring and evaluation data originated. The site could contain links to data related to the benefits of vaccines to support user-friendly navigation.

Scientific independence from other parts of CDC and other relevant government agencies, such as FDA, need not isolate the staff of the vaccine risk monitoring and evaluation office from needed scientific expertise. Consultation and collaboration ought to be fostered, but the final decision making about monitoring and evaluation of vaccine risk information and the scientific content of risk communications needs to remain with this office.

Adhering to the principles behind the other recommendations in this report would support the prompt publication of all risk evaluation information, including null or uncertain findings. While the committee understands the need for quality assurance of research data and peer review, it heard in public comments (see Box 1-5) and key informant interviews (see Appendix C) that publication is sometimes delayed due to burdens of review and CDC clearance. It is important for engendering trust in the safety of vaccines that research results are not perceived as being constrained or hidden. The vaccine risk monitoring and evaluation efforts during the COVID PHE demonstrated that frequent, complete, and timely communications (Gee, 2024; Jernigan, 2025) *can* occur, and the committee thinks speed, completeness, and transparency ought to govern those about vaccine risks. As per this recommendation, CDC should assure that the technical content of these communications is under the purview of the vaccine risk scientists and that clearance of the technical information by offices that promote vaccination ought to be limited to "notification only."

PUBLIC HEALTH EMERGENCIES

The need for relevant vaccine risk information is heightened during a PHE, and it is imperative that health professionals, policy makers, and the public believe the information provided to them. Federal staff doing vaccine risk monitoring, evaluation, and communications can continue to be guided by the principles of relevance, credibility, data stewardship, continual improvement and innovation, and scientific independence detailed earlier, regardless of temporary or situational placement within a whole of government response.

The strategic plan, discussed in relation to Recommendation 1, should include a section on operations during a PHE and plans for an intensive vaccine risk evaluation apparatus, such as the VaST used during the COVID PHE or the processes established during the H1N1 pandemic in 2009 (Markowitz et al., 2024; Yih et al., 2012). A continuity of operations plan would define what routine vaccine risk monitoring, evaluation, and communication work will continue and what will pause, what resources will be shifted to address the emergency, and how risk information will be shared. The emergency plan ought to also include steps for the vaccine risk monitoring and evaluation office to rapidly return to its pre-emergency administrative placement, research agenda, and scientific independence, as soon as possible (Markowitz et al., 2024; Yih et al., 2012).

CONCLUDING THOUGHTS

The committee has concluded that ISO functions well and merits the nation's trust; however, federal vaccine risk monitoring, evaluation, and communication could be enhanced by adhering to the offered set of five recommendations. Implementing these will require resources but also the commitment of the CDC director to protect the office in order to significantly enhance the capability to deliver timely, trustworthy, and scientifically robust vaccine risk information. This, in turn, supports increased public confidence in vaccination programs, ultimately contributing to stronger public health outcomes and preparedness for future public health emergencies.

REFERENCES

CDC (Centers for Disease Control and Prevention). n.d. *How to Access Data from the Vaccine Safety Datalink*. https://archive.cdc.gov/www_cdc_gov/vaccinesafety/ensuringsafety/monitoring/vsd/accessing-data.html (accessed June 5, 2025).

CDC. 2004. *Blue Ribbon Panel Meeting Summary Report June 3 and 4, 2004*. http:/www.cdc.gov/od/ads/brpr/brprsumm.htm#appendix1 (archived April 28, 2005 using the Wayback Machine: https://web.archive.org/web/20060620191520/).

CDC. 2006. *Advisory Committee on Immunization Practices Record of the Proceedings*. https:/www.cdc.gov/vaccines/acip/meetings/downloads/min-archive/min-2006-06-508.pdf (archived March 8, 2021 using the Wayback Machine: https://web.archive.org/web/20210308230331/).

CDC. 2011. *ISO scientific agenda*. https://archive.cdc.gov/www_cdc_gov/vaccinesafety/research/isoscientificagenda/index.html (accessed July 23, 2025).

CDC. 2023. *Emergency Preparedness and Vaccine Safety*. https:/www.cdc.gov/vaccinesafety/ensuringsafety/monitoring/emergencypreparedness/index.html#anchor_1607961664745 (archived May 25, 2024 using the Wayback Machine: https://web.archive.org/web/20240525205459/).

CDC. 2024. *The Federal Statistical System*. https://www.cdc.gov/nchs/about/federal-statistical-system.html (accessed June 4, 2025).

Gee, J. 2024. CDC response to vaccine safety needs for the U.S. COVID-19 vaccination program—an overview of vaccine safety systems. Presentation to the Committee to Review the Centers for Disease Control and Prevention's COVID-19 Vaccine Safety Research and Communications, Washington, DC, August 7.

IOM (Institute of Medicine). 2005. *Vaccine safety research, data access, and public trust.* Washington, DC: The National Academies Press.

ISPE (International Society for Pharmacoepidemiology). 2015. *Guidelines for Good Pharmacoepidemiology Practices (GPP).* https://www.pharmacoepi.org/resources/policies/guidelines-08027/ (accessed June 5, 2025).

ISPE. 2025. *Author Guidelines.* https://onlinelibrary.wiley.com/page/journal/10991557/homepage/forauthors.html (accessed June 5, 2025).

Jernigan, D. 2025. CDC COVID-19 vaccine safety risk communications. Presentation to the Committee to Review the Centers for Disease Control and Prevention's COVID-19 Vaccine Safety Research and Communications, Washington, DC, January 10, 2025.

Markowitz, L. E., R. H. Hopkins Jr, K. R. Broder, G. M. Lee, K. M. Edwards, M. F. Daley, L. A. Jackson, J. C. Nelson, L. E. Riley, and V. V. McNally. 2024. COVID-19 Vaccine Safety Technical (VaST) Work Group: Enhancing vaccine safety monitoring during the pandemic. *Vaccine* 42:125549. https://doi.org/10.1016/j.vaccine.2023.12.059.

NASEM (National Academies of Sciences, Engineering, and Medicine). 2025. *Principles and practices for a federal statistical agency: Eighth edition.* Washington, DC: The National Academies Press.

NIH (National Institutes of Health). 2025. *Protocol Registration Data Element Definitions for Interventional and Observational Studies.* https://clinicaltrials.gov/policy/protocol-definitions#intro (accessed July 9, 2025).

Salmon, D. A., L. H. Moulton, and N. A. Halsey. 2004. Enhancing public confidence in vaccines through independent oversight of postlicensure vaccine safety. *American Journal of Public Health* 94(6):947–950. https://doi.org/10.2105/AJPH.94.6.947.

VAERS (Vaccine Adverse Event Reporting System). n.d. *VAERS Data.* https://vaers.hhs.gov/data.html (accessed June 5, 2025).

Yih, W. K., G. M. Lee, T. A. Lieu, R. Ball, M. Kulldorff, M. Rett, P. M. Wahl, C. N. McMahill-Walraven, R. Platt, and D. A. Salmon. 2012. Surveillance for adverse events following receipt of pandemic 2009 H1N1 vaccine in the Post-Licensure Rapid Immunization Safety Monitoring (PRISM) system, 2009–2010. *American Journal of Epidemiology* 175(11):1120–1128. https://doi.org/10.1093/aje/kws197.

Appendix A

Committee Member and Staff Biographies

COMMITTEE MEMBER BIOGRAPHIES

Jane E. Henney, M.D., has had a distinguished career in academia, government service, and the governance of both corporate and not-for-profit organizations. Her government service began at the National Cancer Institute (NCI), where she served as deputy director. She was deputy commissioner for operations at the Food and Drug Administration (FDA) and in 1998 was confirmed as Commissioner. She has led two major public academic health centers: the University of New Mexico and the University of Cincinnati. She was elected to National Academy of Medicine (NAM) membership in 2000. She has chaired several consensus studies and served on and chaired the NAM Membership Committee. In 2014, she was appointed as NAM Home Secretary and in 2018 was the first elected home secretary, serving until 2020. Dr. Henney received her M.D. in 1973 from Indiana University School of Medicine, and her training in oncology was completed at M.D. Anderson and NCI. She served on the Board of AmerisourceBergen and has residual financial holdings from this role. She was the chair of the University of Kansas Advancement Committee.

Denise H. Crysler, J.D., served as the director of the Network for Public Health Law's Mid-States Region for over 12 years. She recently retired from this position and now serves as a senior advisor to the network. Through the network, she worked on the IZ Gateway project, a Centers for Disease Control and Prevention-funded effort that facilitates exchange of immunization information with immunization information systems. Before joining the network, Ms. Chrysler provided legal services to Michigan's state health department regarding communicable disease, immunization, environmental public health, public health research, privacy, health information exchange, and emergency legal preparedness and response. She received the 2019 Roy J. Manty Distinguished Service Award for contributions to public health in Michigan. Ms. Chrysler previously served on her local board of health and was cochair of the Public Health Law Subcommittee of the Council of State and Territorial Epidemiologists. She also served on the National Committee on Vital and Health Statistics. Ms. Chrysler graduated from the University of Michigan Law School and is a licensed attorney in Michigan.

Lawrence Deyton, M.S.P.H., M.D., is the Murdock Head Professor of Medicine and Health Policy and, from 2014 until July 1, 2023, was the senior associate dean for clinical public health at the George Washington (GW) University's School of Medicine and Health Sciences. Before joining the GW faculty in 2014, he served in leadership positions at several federal agencies, including as the founding director of the Center for Tobacco Products at the Food and Drug Administration (FDA). Prior to joining FDA, Dr. Deyton held several leadership positions at the Department of Veterans Affairs (VA). He oversaw VA's public health programs, including environmental hazards and public health surveillance programs, women's health, occupational health, and emergency preparedness and responses of VA's health system. In 2019, he received the James Bruce Award for Distinguished Contributions in Preventive Medicine by the American College of Physicians. He earned his M.D. from the George Washington University School of Medicine and M.S.P.H. at the Harvard School of Public Health. Dr. Deyton has served on several National Academies of Sciences, Engineering, and Medicine (National Academies) studies.

Francisco García, M.D., M.P.H., is the chief of staff to the president of the University of Arizona and a professor emeritus of public health. Until January of 2025, he was the deputy county administrator and chief medical officer for Pima County, Arizona, where he oversaw the departments of Health, Behavioral Health, Environmental Quality; Pima Animal Care Center; Community & Workforce Development; offices of Emergency Management, Medical Examiner, and Digital Equity; and the Pima County Libraries. Prior to entering government in 2013, Dr. García was a tenured distinguished outreach professor of obstetrics and gynecology and public health. He served in a variety of leadership roles, including as the director of the University of Arizona Center of Excellence in Women's Health, chair of the Section of Family and Child Health of the Mel & Enid Zuckerman College of Public Health, and director of the Cancer Disparities Institute of the Arizona Cancer Center. Dr. García was elected to NAM in 2023. He has served on the National Academies Committee on Evidence-Based Practices for Public Health Emergency Preparedness and Response, Roundtable on Health Equity, and Committee on Preventive Services for Women. He is a former member of the U.S. Preventive Services Task Force. He received an M.D. from the University of Arizona and M.P.H. from Johns Hopkins University.

Krishika Graham, M.D., M.P.H., is the unit chief for vaccine-preventable disease surveillance with the New York City (NYC) Department of Health and Mental Hygiene's Bureau of Immunization. The bureau receives funding from the Centers for Disease Control and Prevention to support coordination for enhanced vaccine-preventable and respiratory diseases surveillance. She has served as the vaccine safety branch director during NYC's monkeypox outbreak response, leading an evaluation of vaccine reactogenicity and safety of Jynneos vaccine using a survey of vaccine recipients in New York City's immunization registry during a period of expanded use. She also led outreach and enrollment of Federally Qualified Health Centers and independent pharmacies in the NYC COVID-19 Vaccine Program. She is a board-certified pediatrician and preventive medicine physician. She received her M.D. from the University of Virginia and M.P.H. from the CUNY Graduate School of Public Health & Health Policy.

Marie Griffin, M.D., M.P.H., is professor of health policy, emerita at Vanderbilt University School of Medicine. Her research focused on the safety and effectiveness of drugs and vaccines, and the burden of vaccine-preventable diseases. She developed novel methods to quantify the medical care burden of common respiratory viruses in both children and adults. Dr. Griffin recently served on the National Institute of Allergy and Infectious Diseases Data and Safety Monitoring Committee for COVID-19 Vaccine Clinical Trials. She is a member of the FDA's Drug Safety and Risk Management Advisory Committee and CDC Advisory Committee on Immunization Practices work group on RSV vaccines. She is vice-chair of the Metro Nashville Board of Health. Dr. Griffin is the recipient Grant W. Liddle Award for Outstanding Contributions to Research at Vanderbilt University Medical Center, Association for Clinical and Translational Science Distinguished Investigator Award for Translation from Clinical Use into Public Benefit and Policy, Mary Jane Werthan Award for Advancement of Women at Vanderbilt, and Elaine Sanders-Bush Award for Mentoring Graduate and/or Medical Students in Research Settings at Vanderbilt. Dr. Griffin has served on National Academies committees relating to vaccine safety. She received her M.P.H. from Johns Hopkins School of Hygiene and Public Health and M.D. from Georgetown University Medical School.

Perry N. Halkitis, Ph.D., is dean, Hunterdon Professor of Public Health & Health Equity, and Distinguished Professor of Biostatistics & Epidemiology at the Rutgers School of Public Health. He is an infectious disease epidemiologist, applied statistician, and public health psychologist. For 3 decades, the focus of his research has been on the emergence, prevention, and treatment of infectious diseases in sexual, gender, and/or racial and ethnic minority populations. He is the founder and director of the Center for Health, Identity, Behavior & Prevention Studies. He is professor emeritus at the College of Global Public Health at New York University. He is an elected fellow of the New York Academy of Medicine, The Society of Behavioral Medicine, The American Epidemiological Society, The European Academy of Translational Medicine, College of Physicians of Philadelphia, and four divisions of the American Psychological Association. He is the editor in chief of *Behavioral Medicine* since 2013 and founding editor in chief of *Annals of LGBTQ Public and Population Health*. Dr. Halkitis serves on the board of directors of the Association for School and Programs of Public Health (as chair in 2023–2024) and Hyacinth Foundation. He also serves on the advisory boards of both the New Jersey Public Health Advisory Committee and the Behavioral Risk Factor Survey Advisory Committee. Dr. Halkitis holds degrees in epidemiology, applied statistics, psychology, and education from the City University of New York.

Sonia Hernández-Díaz, M.D., Dr.P.H., is professor of epidemiology at the Harvard T.H. Chan School of Public Health, where she serves as director of the Pharmacoepidemiology & Real-World Evidence Program. Her research focuses on examining the safety of pharmaceuticals using observational data, with a special interest on pregnant women and their infants. Another group of research activities concerns the application of innovative methodologic concepts to increase the validity of nonrandomized studies. She helped develop methods for emulating trials to evaluate the effectiveness and safety of COVID vaccines during pregnancy and collaborated with the COVID-19 Vaccines International Pregnancy Exposure Registry, under the aegis of Preregistry. She receives salary support for work on the Massachusetts General Hospital (MGH) Anti-Epileptic Drugs pregnancy registry funded by multiple pharmaceutical companies, including Janssen. She also serves as a compensated member of the Scientific Committee for the MGH Antipsychotics drug registry. Her research on the effects of constipation drugs on pregnancy is supported by Takeda Pharmaceuticals. She was compensated for providing consulting services to J&J and currently consults for Moderna and Roche for work unrelated to vaccines. Dr. Hernández-Díaz has served as chair for the Drug Safety and Risk Management Advisory Committee of FDA, reviewer for the Eunice Kennedy Shriver National

Institute of Child Health and Human Development Pregnancy & Neonatology Study Section, and member of the Teratogenic Information Services Advisory Board. She was elected president of the Society for Perinatal and Pediatric Epidemiology in 2014 and president of the International Society for Pharmacoepidemiology in 2015. Dr. Hernández-Díaz received her M.D. from the Autonoma University of Madrid Medical School and Dr.P.H. in epidemiology from the Harvard School of Public Health.

Ali S. Khan, M.D., is the Richard Holland Presidential Chair and Dean of the College of Public Health at the University of Nebraska Medical Center. He is a former assistant surgeon general with the U.S. Public Health Service. His career has focused on health security, global health, climate change, and emerging infections. He completed a 23-year career as a senior director at the Centers for Disease Control and Prevention (CDC), where he led and responded to numerous high profile domestic and international public health responses. Dr. Khan was one of the main architects of CDC's national health security program with an early focus on preparations for acquisition and use of smallpox and anthrax vaccines. He frequently speaks about and publishes on improving childhood and adult immunization access and addressing vaccine hesitancy. He is the author of *The Next Pandemic: On the Front Lines Against Humankind's Gravest Dangers*. Dr. Khan has served on several National Academies committees, including the Committee on Best Practices in Assessing Morbidity and Mortality Following Large-Scale Disasters. He received his M.D. from Downstate Medical University, completed a med-peds residency at the University of Michigan, followed by his M.P.H. from Emory University and M.B.A. from University of Nebraska–Omaha.

Daniella Meeker, Ph.D., is an associate professor in the Section of Biomedical Informatics and Data Science and the chief research information Officer at Yale University School of Medicine and Yale New Haven Health System. Dr. Meeker's expertise is in applications of behavioral economics to improve quality of care, analysis of claims and electronic medical record data, and managing large, multi-institutional electronic health record-integrated studies. Dr. Meeker has received the Behavioral Publication Award for Innovation in Behavioral Policy (2019), Scientific Program Committee AMIA (2015), Merkin Scholarship for Neuroscience and Policy (2015), Robert Brook Scholarship Award (2013), and Distinguished Fellow with Roybal Center for Health Policy Simulation (2012). Dr. Meeker received her Ph.D. in Computation and Neural Systems from the California Institute of Technology in Pasadena, CA.

Glen Nowak, Ph.D., is a professor, an Associate Dean for Research and Graduate Studies, and codirector of a Center for Risk & Health Communication in the Grady College of Journalism & Mass Communication at the University of Georgia. He is a national and internationally known expert in health and risk communication research and training related to infectious and vaccine-preventable diseases, crisis, and emergency risk communication and vaccination acceptance and decision making. Before rejoining the University of Georgia (UGA) faculty in January 2013, Dr. Nowak spent 14 years at the Centers for Disease Control and Prevention, including 6 years as the communications director for the National Immunization Program and 6 years as the agency's director of media relations. Dr. Nowak is coeditor of the recently published book *Advancing Crisis Communication Effectiveness*. In the past, he provided presentations on vaccine hesitancy and acceptance in multiple settings, including with a Janssen Advisory Board in 2020. He has served as an expert on issues related to vaccine confidence and safety with the National Vaccine Advisory Committee and Council for Quality Health Communication, among others. Dr. Nowak received his B.S. from the University of Wisconsin–Milwaukee, with majors in economics and communications. He has an M.A. in journalism and a Ph.D. in mass communications from the University of Wisconsin–Madison.

Olayinka Shiyanbola, Ph.D., B.Pharm., is Charles R. Walgreen Jr. Professor in the Department of Clinical Pharmacy at the University of Michigan College of Pharmacy. Dr. Shiyanbola's research examines patient perceptions and roles in medication use and its impact on medication adherence, health literacy and the elimination of health disparities. Specifically, Dr. Shiyanbola studies the perceptions of illness and medicines among marginalized populations. She interweaves patient perspectives into the implementation of tailored patient-centered medication use interventions. She uses sociobehavioral and health psychology theories in her studies and employs qualitative, quantitative, and mixed methods approaches in her work. As a National Institutes of Health scholar/fellow, Dr. Shiyanbola received training in health disparities research, randomized behavioral clinical trials, and mixed methods. She was a Society of Behavioral Medicine Leadership Fellow and is an appointed member of the National Academies Roundtable on Health Literacy. She received her B.Pharm. from the University of Ibadan in Nigeria and Ph.D. in pharmaceutical socioeconomics from the University of Iowa in Iowa City.

Lillie Williamson, Ph.D., is assistant professor in the Department of Communication Arts at the University of Wisconsin—Madison. Dr. Williamson's research broadly examines the ways in which lived experiences intersect with and can influence health communication. Much of her work investigates the interactions between communication within and outside the clinical context and medical mistrust, particularly for Black Americans. Her current projects explore communication about medical racism, shared trust between clinicians and patients, and the creation of community-driven, culturally responsive science communication strategies and messages. Dr. Williamson holds a B.S. in biology and psychology from the University of North Carolina—Chapel Hill and an M.A. and Ph.D. in communication from the University of Illinois—Urbana-Champaign.

STAFF BIOGRAPHIES

Kathleen Stratton, Ph.D., is a scholar in the Health and Medicine Division (HMD) Board on Population Health and Public Health Practice (BPH). She began her career at the National Academies in 1990 in the Institute of Medicine (IOM). She has spent most of her time with the BPH. She has staffed committees addressing vaccine safety and development, pandemic preparedness, environmental and occupational health, drug safety, clinical prevention research, and tobacco control. She was given the IOM Cecil Research Award for sustained contributions to vaccine safety and made a staff scholar in 2005. She received a B.A. in natural sciences from Johns Hopkins University and a Ph.D. in pharmacology and toxicology from the University of Maryland at Baltimore.

Ogan Kumova, Ph.D., is a program officer at the National Academies in HMD. He was a research fellow at the Food and Drug Administration's (FDA) Office of Vaccine Research and Review, where he worked on developing vaccines for infectious diseases. During his time at FDA, Dr. Kumova was a coinvestigator on grants evaluating the safety and immunogenicity of vaccine adjuvants and developing vaccines for meningococcal and gonococcal infections. He obtained his Ph.D. in immunology from Drexel University College of Medicine in Philadelphia, Pennsylvania. In his graduate work, Dr. Kumova studied neonatal immune responses and modifiable risk factors for respiratory viral infections and collaborated with several labs, including Wistar Cancer Institute, to develop DNA-based HIV vaccines. He holds a B.S. in biochemistry and bioinformatics from the University of the Sciences in Philadelphia and an M.S. in clinical infectious diseases from Drexel University.

Dara Ancona, M.P.H., is an associate program officer in the Health and Medicine Division on the Board on Population Health and Public Health Practice. Before joining the National Academies, Mrs. Ancona was an epidemiologist at a local health department. She has experience with communicable disease investigations, public health emergency preparedness, and data analysis, specifically with STI/HIV and COVID data. She completed her B.S. in health sciences at New York Institute of Technology and M.P.H. in epidemiology from George Washington University.

Katie Peterson is a senior program assistant in the Health and Medicine Division. Ms. Peterson supports consensus studies on public health topics of vaccine communications and military health. She graduated from Purdue University, where she double majored in women's, gender, and sexuality studies and anthropology. She concentrated in applied anthropology, anthropology of health, and cultural anthropology. Additionally, she earned minors in psychology and French.

Olivia Loibner was a senior program assistant in the Health and Medicine Division until August 2024. She contributed to studies and workshops on a variety of public health topics, including the Review of Relevant Literature of Adverse Effects Associated with Vaccines, the Review of the Department of VA Presumption Decision Process, and others. Ms. Loibner graduated from American University with a B.A. in international studies.

Rose Marie Martinez, Sc.D., has been the senior board director of the Board on Population Health and Public Health Practice (BPH) since 1999. BPH addresses the science base for population health and public health interventions and examines the capacity of the health system, particularly the public health infrastructure, to support disease prevention and health promotion activities, including the education and supply of health professionals necessary for carrying them out. BPH has examined such topics as the safety of childhood vaccines and other drugs, systems for evaluating and ensuring drug safety post-marketing, the health effects of cannabis and cannabinoids, the health effects of environmental exposures, population health improvement strategies, the integration of medical care and public health, women's health services, health disparities, health literacy, tobacco control strategies, and chronic disease prevention, among others. Dr. Martinez was awarded the 2010 IOM Research Cecil Award for significant contributions to IOM reports of exceptional quality and influence. Before joining the National Academies, Dr. Martinez was a senior health researcher at Mathematica Policy Research (1995–1999), where she conducted research on the impact of health system change on public health infrastructure, access to care for vulnerable populations, managed care, and the health care workforce. Dr. Martinez is a former assistant director for health financing and policy with the U.S. General Accountability Office, where she directed evaluations and policy analysis in the area of national and public health issues (1988–1995). Her experience also includes 6 years directing research studies for the Regional Health Ministry of Madrid, Spain (1982–1988). Dr. Martinez is a member of the Council on Education for Public Health, the accreditation body for schools of public health and public health programs. She received the degree of Doctor of Science from the Johns Hopkins School of Hygiene and Public Health.

Appendix B

Public Meeting Agendas for the Committee to Review the Center for Disease Control and Prevention's COVID-19 Vaccine Safety Research and Communications

FIRST INFORMATION GATHERING SESSION
June 24, 2024
Washington, DC

1:00	Welcome and Introductions; Conduct of the Open Session *Jane Henney, M.D., Committee Chair*
1:00–2:30	Presentation by CDC Immunization Safety Office on the Statement of Task *John Su, M.D., Acting Director, Immunization Safety Office (virtual)* Q&A with Committee *John Su, M.D., Acting Director, Immunization Safety Office (virtual)*
2:30	**Closing Comments, OPEN SESSION ENDS** *Jane Henney, M.D., Committee Chair*

SECOND INFORMATION GATHERING SESSION
August 7, 2024
Washington, DC

2:00	Welcome and Introductions; Conduct of the Open Session *Jane Henney, M.D., Committee Chair*
2:00–4:00	CDC Response to Vaccines Safety Needs for the U.S. COVID-19 Vaccination Program: An Overview of Vaccine Safety Systems *Julianne Gee, MPH, Senior Advisor, ISO, CDC (virtual)*
4:00	Closing Remarks, OPEN SESSION ENDS *Jane Henney, M.D., Committee Chair*

THIRD INFORMATION GATHERING SESSION
October 11, 2024

Virtual

11:00-11:10	Welcome and Introductions; Conduct of the Public Comment Session *Jane Henney, M.D., Committee Chair*
11:00–1:00	The Committee to Review the Centers for Disease Control and Prevention's COVID-19 Vaccine Safety Research and Communications Public Comment Session
1:00	Closing Remarks, OPEN SESSION ENDS *Jane Henney, M.D., Committee Chair*

FOURTH INFORMATION GATHERING SESSION
January 10, 2025

Washington, DC

10:30	Welcome and Introductions; Conduct of the Public Comment Session *Jane Henney, M.D., Committee Chair*

APPENDIX B   123

10:30–12:30   Presentation on CDC COVID-19 Vaccine Safety Risk
              Communications
              *Daniel Jernigan, M.D., MPH, Director, National
              Center for Emerging and Zoonotic Infectious Diseases
              (NCEZID) (virtual)*

12:30   Closing Remarks, OPEN SESSION ENDS
              Jane Henney, M.D., Committee Chair

FIFTH INFORMATION GATHERING SESSION
February 25, 2025

Washington, DC

1:00   Welcome and Introductions; Conduct of the Public
              Comment Session
              Jane Henney, M.D., Committee Chair

1:00–2:30   Presentation on Challenges and Opportunities for
              Research and Communication About Vaccine Safety
              *Reed Tuckson, M.D., Tuckson Health Connections, LLC,
              Black Coalition Against COVID*

              *Lisa Fitzgerald, M.D., MPH, MPA, Grapevine Health
              (Unable to attend)*

              Malia Jones, Ph.D., University of Wisconsin, Madison

              *Scott Razan, M.D., MPA, M.A., CUNY Graduate School
              of Public Health & Health Policy*

2:30   Closing Remarks, OPEN SESSION ENDS
              Jane Henney, M.D., Committee Chair

Appendix C

Westat Key Informant Interviews Findings Report
Support to the NASEM Review of CDC COVID-19 Vaccine Safety Research and Communications

May 30, 2025

Authors:

Jennifer Edwards, Neni Osuoha, Jennifer Maizel, Rachel Neenan, Nina Page, Paul Reischmann, Beth Slotman

This study was conducted by Westat with the National Academy of Sciences. The findings and conclusions in this report are those of the authors and should not be construed to represent any official NASEM determination or policy.

CONTENTS

A.	Background	127
B.	Study Design	127
	Sample	127
	Recruitment and Data Collection	129
	Interviews	130
	Analysis	131
C.	Findings: Cross-Cutting Themes	132
	Infrastructure, Resources, and Processes	132
	Coordination and Collaboration	135
	Communications	138
D.	Findings: Distinct Themes by Group	141
	CDC VSD Sites	141
	CDC-Funded Researchers: CISA	142
	Healthcare Professionals	145
	Vaccine Safety Experts	147
	State and Local Public Health Officials	149
E.	Conclusions	152
	Study Limitations	152
	Overarching Findings	153

Appendix A. Interview Guides	155
Appendix B. Recruitment Letters	172
Appendix C. Informed Consent	175

A. BACKGROUND

The National Academies of Sciences, Engineering and Medicine (NASEM) Health and Medicine Division tasked Westat with supporting a consensus study evaluating the Centers for Disease Control and Prevention (CDC) Immunization Safety Office (ISO) systems, methods, and processes for monitoring COVID-19 vaccine safety during the U.S. COVID-19 public health emergency (PHE). This study aimed to identify recommendations for sustaining, maintaining, and strengthening CDC ISO's monitoring systems and communications moving forward.

Westat was responsible for conducting confidential key informant interviews with a wide array of individuals who have direct experience and knowledge of CDC ISO efforts. These interviews solicited perspectives on ISO's processes, research, and communications about COVID-19 vaccine safety during the COVID-19 public health emergency (PHE), interagency and cross- sector collaboration, successes and challenges during the PHE, and recommendations for process improvements. This report summarizes key themes found across these interviews.

B. STUDY DESIGN

Sample

The NASEM Committee appointed to conduct the overarching study, supported by NASEM staff, identified several categories of key informants relevant to this qualitative study: CDC ISO staff, staff from other CDC offices, staff from other federal agencies, CDC-funded researchers from Vaccine Safety Datalink (VSD) sites and the Clinical Immunization Safety Assessment (CISA) program, external vaccine safety experts (VSEs), healthcare professionals (HCPs), and public health officials (PHOs). NASEM staff compiled lists of potential participants from these groups who in effect served as the population of interest for this study. Sources of information for developing these lists included the ISO Directory, Advisory Committee on Immunization Practices (ACIP) current and former members and ex-officio representatives, publications and public information, and Committee recommendations.

Key Informant Interview Groups

The Westat team developed a sample design with targets for each identified key informant group; however, recruitment proved to be challenging, precluding reaching these targets for most groups.

Table 1 provides a summary of the key informant groups invited to participate and the number of interviews across each group that were completed. In late January 2025, the Department of Health and Human Services instructed staff to pause external public health communications.

Out of an abundance of caution, ISO directed a pause on proceeding with interviews of CDC staff. As a result, this group had to be excluded. Some interviews were with multiple participants; for example, VSD site interviews typically involved two participants. Additionally, one interview with VSEs, originally planned as a focus group, had only two participants. In this instance, we made an effort to provide each respondent with an opportunity to answer each interview question separately.

In the case of non-ISO CDC staff and other federal agency staff, we received responses from one former CDC employee, one National Institutes of Health (NIH) employee, and one Food and Drug Administration (FDA) employee. These three interviews were grouped together as "other federal staff." However, given that each participant came from distinct offices and agencies with different roles, the findings from this group essentially present three distinct perspectives. We discuss how these perspectives were integrated into our thematic analysis in the following sections.

Table 1. Key Informant Interview Group Categories

Group		Initial sample	Completed
CDC	ISO	65	0
	Other	6	1
Other feds		20	2
CDC-funded researchers	VSD	16	7*
	CISA	8	5
HCP		44	4
VSE		29	6
Public health officials	State	11	2
	Local	74	3
	Tribal	15	0
Totals		288	30

*7 VSD sites participated in interviews

APPENDIX C

NOTE: Several participants had multiple identities and professional experiences influencing their perspectives (e.g., physician and PH official).

Recruitment and Data Collection

Introductory Emails

To encourage participation, ISO and NASEM sent out initial emails to the participant pool to inform them of the study and advise them of Westat's pending invitation to participate. Once this occurred, Westat sent individual emails to key informants inviting their participation; these emails included a link to a brief Qualtrics survey and information regarding interview scheduling, which are described below. Some of the emails were unique in that two individuals that worked together in the CDC-funded research group were sent a joint email to schedule a meeting together.

Westat's outreach emails were sent on three different occasions, approximately one week apart to increase engagement. We also followed up individually with potential participants who noted interest in the survey but did not schedule an interview.

Qualtrics Survey

Westat created a recruitment survey administered via Qualtrics, a FedRAMP-compliant and secure online platform. The survey was sent to all potential participants as a tool to signal their interest in participating in the study, confirm their role or type of key informant group during the PHE, and collect their preferred method of contact and form of participation (individual interview or focus group). Additionally, the survey asked questions (some of which were optional) pertaining to a participant's general professional information, such as their current role/area(s) of expertise, their office/agency/institution, and their familiarity with different vaccine safety systems.

In total, 69 survey responses were received. In addition, a participant who did not fill out the survey sent an email to signal interest.

Interview Scheduling

To schedule interviews, we sent out links via Calendly, an online meeting scheduling app, that provided participants the opportunity to select a time that worked for them. Of the 69 individuals who completed the Qualtrics survey, seven noted at this time that they no longer wanted to participate, and 11 were in the CDC ISO group. Of the remaining individuals who expressed an interest in completing interviews, three canceled their interviews, one did not show up to their interview, and 17 did not respond to interview scheduling requests.

Interviews

All interviews were held via Zoom. Individual interviews lasted approximately 60 minutes and our one small-group interview lasted approximately 90 minutes. Interviews were semi-structured; Westat developed a set of core interview questions for each key informant group based on Committee questions and research aims (see Appendix A), and additional probes or follow-up questions were asked as needed and based on informants' unique responses. The interview questions spanned an array of topics related to vaccine safety research processes, agency/institutional collaborations, resources, infrastructures, leadership, communications, and others. Some topics were cross-cutting and asked of multiple key informant groups, while other topics were only applicable to one group.

Cross-Cutting Topics

- Relationship with/perceptions of CDC ISO
- Sufficiency of vaccine safety resources and systems
- CDC vaccine safety communications, public perception, and influence
- General experience during the PHE, suggestions for improvement at ISO

Group-Specific Topics

- Researchers: Vaccine safety research priorities and independence
- Other federal agency staff: Resource allocation, coordination in federal vaccine safety efforts
- Healthcare professionals (HCPs): Use of CDC vaccine safety systems
- External vaccine safety experts (VSEs): Use of CDC data and collaborations
- Public health officials (PHOs): Vaccine safety information access/adaptation

Topics Not Able to Be Addressed

The Committee expressed interest in and developed questions on staffing and reporting structures within ISO during the PHE, ISO organizational issues, intra-CDC coordination, and the impact of ISO's placement within CDC. These questions were unique to CDC staff and ISO. Because we were unable to interview this key informant group, these topics could not be addressed. Additionally, questions around resource sufficiency were generally answered by other key informant groups at a macro level, and they provided limited insight on post-PHE changes.

Analysis

We interpreted participant's responses using an iterative, multistep process of coding, analysis, and synthesis of findings. Team members were divided by key informant groups for each step.

Codebook Development

As we neared the end of data collection, the team collaborated on developing a codebook for both structural and thematic analysis based on insights collected from the interviews. The codebook was designed to be broadly applicable and capture information at a high level across key informant groups. It included structural codes based on interview topics and thematic codes that captured distinct issues specific to key informant groups. Not all codes were relevant for all key informant groups, though some codes were comprehensive, capturing the perspectives of multiple key informant groups.

NVivo Analysis

We uploaded interview transcripts[1] to NVivo, a qualitative data analysis program, to conduct structural coding based on interview topics and thematic coding for specific concepts that were discussed. Transcripts were organized in NVivo using case classifications, which categorized transcripts by key informant groups.

Team members reviewed interview transcripts to code potential findings according to the codebook and were encouraged to use annotations to note any specific details for further analysis during the synthesis phase. For a consistent and reliable application of the codebook, all team

---

[1] Interviews were transcribed by Rev.com unless the participant requested not to be recorded. In those handful of cases, a second researcher participated in the interview to note-taking purposes.

members first coded the same transcript and discussed which codes could use further specificity or a refined definition. Once completed, the remaining transcripts were divided among the team for individual coding. Team members met on a weekly basis to ask questions and discuss preliminary findings during the coding process.

Synthesis of Findings

Once all coding was completed, the team used NVivo to run queries of the codes and annotations of interview transcripts to generate coding results (i.e., all the information coded to a specific topic and key informant group). Team members first reviewed the coding results for each key informant group, identifying reoccurring themes and shared perspectives within groups as well as outlier perspectives. Then the team met to determine whether themes emerging for a specific key informant group overlapped with themes that came up in other key informant groups. Themes that overlapped with more than one key informant group were considered cross-cutting, and themes that were distinct to one key informant group were considered group-specific.

C. FINDINGS: CROSS-CUTTING THEMES

Cross-cutting themes were categorized into three general thematic areas: (1) Infrastructure, Resources, and Processes; (2) Coordination and Collaboration; and (3) Communication.

Infrastructure, Resources, and Processes

All participants were asked to describe the sufficiency of ISO's and the existing vaccine safety systems' infrastructure, resources, and processes during the COVID-19 PHE. As mentioned above, the study team's inability to interview CDC and ISO staff members meant that some facets of ISO's infrastructure, including reporting structures, internal organization and processes, and the influence of ISO's placement within CDC, could not be investigated. Participants across all groups shared strong positive reactions to the increase in resources and processes put in place in response to the PHE, as well as ISO leaders' qualifications and strong response to the pressures of the PHE. However, researchers and VSEs shared that even this bolstered infrastructure was still insufficient in several ways during the PHE, and they shared several suggestions for developing an infrastructure better prepared for future crises.

Successes

Increased resources and funding during the PHE

Multiple groups reported increased resources and funding allocated toward vaccine safety during the PHE, and these increases facilitated strong research and an effective PHE response. All federal agency staff felt they had the resources needed to ramp up vaccine safety efforts during the PHE (e.g., due to additional funding, they had the ability to hire more staff). A few CISA and VSD researchers also felt that the influx of funding and staffing facilitated an effective emergency response.

Effective structures and processes during the PHE

Multiple groups described successes tied to the structures and processes of federal vaccine safety systems. All federal agency staff agreed that established processes at CDC, the FDA, and other agencies worked well during the PHE, and that what changed the most was the frequency, intensity, and/or speed of work. These participants noted the value and importance of already having the systems, relationships, and communication mechanisms in place to enable what they saw as a successful response to the PHE. All CISA researchers noted that the existing infrastructure and relationships within CISA and between CISA and ISO enabled effective clinical and research responses. A few CISA researchers specifically mentioned the effectiveness of the co–principal investigator structure that prepared each CISA institution for the eventual retirement of its "founding principal investigator" (PI) by training their successor on the job through co-PI status. All VSD researchers thought the infrastructure and contract structure of VSD facilitated rapid and responsive research during the PHE.

Two federal agency staff also noted that new vaccine safety study protocols and tools developed during the PHE (e.g., V-safe) have had a lasting impact, as they are being adapted for other needs and can help with future PHE preparedness.

Effective leadership during the PHE

Several groups indicated that CDC ISO "did the best they could" with the vaccine safety resources they had available during the PHE. Most VSD researchers noted CDC ISO leadership (and specifically, the CDC

ISO director and VSD lead) was effective and collaborative during the PHE. Most CISA researchers also spoke highly of ISO leadership during the PHE, for example, noting their effectiveness at navigating bureaucracy, fostering a collaborative spirit, and mobilizing resources. One CISA researcher praised ISO's pandemic-era CISA Team Leader for her outstanding capacity to expedite project launches despite bureaucratic hurdles.

Challenges
Additional resources and infrastructure were needed during the PHE

Despite the robust existing vaccine safety infrastructure and the increased resources and funding during the PHE, most groups stated that these were still insufficient, and more resources and funding were needed.

All CISA researchers and most VSEs noted that CISA's funding, prioritization, and awareness- building resources were insufficient. VSEs noted that CISA particularly lacked the infrastructure for adverse event follow-up. Most VSEs also thought that VSD was limited by its size and funding, and half the VSEs felt V-safe had insufficient infrastructure to support adverse event follow-up.

Although they viewed VSD's database as large, a few VSEs noted it did not have enough data to stratify adverse events by subpopulations. Additionally, one VSE described challenges gaining access to VSD's data, which needed to be provided by the VSD team.

Recommendations
More proactive systems supported and sustained by a robust infrastructure

All external VSEs and some CISA researchers called for a more proactive and robust vaccine safety infrastructure, including more funding, resources, and adverse event follow-up efforts. All VSEs advocated for increased and sustained funding and resources put toward vaccine safety systems and research. A few CISA researchers suggested that the infrastructure developed during the PHE needs to be used more proactively, rather than reactively, to prepare for potential future pandemics; notably, by maintaining communication channels between researchers and frontline providers that were developed during the PHE and leveraging the large groups of researchers and experts brought together for clinical consultations during the PHE to anticipate and study future vaccine safety questions.

Coordination and Collaboration

Interview protocols for VSD and CISA researchers and other VSEs included questions exploring how successful or challenging it was to work with CDC during the COVID-19 PHE. Because of this, findings on coordination and collaboration primarily reflect the perspectives of these research-focused groups and cannot be generalized to other key informant groups or entities. Overall, interviewees shared mostly positive experiences collaborating with CDC on vaccine safety research. However, some researchers encountered challenges and delays in CDC approval and publishing processes, which also posed potential risks to their research independence. Notably, VSD and CISA researchers shared conflicting perspectives on whether their level of input into research priorities was sufficient for effective collaboration. Based on interviewees' feedback, recommendations to improve coordination and collaboration include reducing barriers to CDC's approval and publishing of research, and enhanced coordination between CDC and other federal agencies.

Successes

Effective partnerships between CDC and other researchers

Interviewees across several groups described positive experiences working with CDC staff. Nearly all VSD researchers and federal agency staff characterized their relationship with CDC as a collaborative and respectful partnership. Some VSEs echoed this sentiment, noting that ISO staff were responsive to their questions and keen to share information. Most CISA researchers felt that the ISO team demonstrated strong leadership and communications skills during the PHE, developed positive and productive relationships with contracted researchers, and were effective in establishing the infrastructure and administrative support needed to sustain CISA research and clinical consideration activities.

Challenges

Delays and barriers in research publishing and approval processes

Most VSD and CISA researchers, and a few VSEs, described challenges with CDC's research clearance and publishing processes. They noted that the review process could be slow and cumbersome, sometimes delaying the distribution of time-sensitive research findings. A few VSD researchers thought there were too many separate rounds of review, or that the clearance process included reviewers who did not have appropriate expertise to effectively and efficiently review manuscripts. One VSE described an experience in which concerns regarding potential Freedom of Information Act (FOIA) requests significantly delayed their research being published.

While most interviewees' concerns pertained to clearance and review processes, some researchers also described barriers related to award and approval processes. Most CISA researchers agreed that the yearly timeline for proposal awards is too slow and too rigid, preventing researchers from studying quick-turnaround events such as seasonal vaccine administrations.

Potential risks to research independence during the publishing process

A few VSD researchers described scenarios during the PHE in which CDC reviewers suggested changes that the VSD researchers did not agree with during the clearance process. In two of these cases, researchers perceived that the issue stemmed from reviewers lacking adequate expertise to understand and interpret the study design and findings. One of these researchers noted they were able to provide input to ensure CDC communications about the study accurately reflected its findings, while another researcher explained that they were unsure how to get their publication cleared without having to accept the edits that they disagreed with.

Another VSD researcher shared an instance in which CDC reviewers outside of ISO wanted to highlight and overstate a potential vaccine benefit identified in their study. The researchers who conducted the study believed the finding of this potential vaccine benefit was untrue and likely resulting from bias, and they strongly disagreed with any mention of potential vaccine benefits when the study was designed to assess vaccine safety risks. The researchers involved had to repeatedly emphasize and explain this distinction to CDC staff throughout the clearance process to ensure communications about their study stayed accurate. One VSE also noted challenges and delays tied to cooperative agreements requiring CDC staff to coauthor publications with them, since this requires their research to be vetted by government clearance processes and reduces scientific independence. They noted this contrasts with NIH, which does not require NIH staff to coauthor publications.

Mixed Perspectives

Level of involvement in setting research priorities

VSD and CISA researchers held contrasting views regarding their involvement throughout the research process, particularly in setting research priorities. All VSD researchers noted they were able to provide input on research priorities and propose vaccine safety studies. They described the research priority setting as a collaborative and iterative process with CDC rather than a hierarchy in which CDC would have given rigid task orders to researchers. A few CISA researchers shared this perspective and noted that they were involved to some extent in priority setting.

However, most CISA researchers wished that they could have been included earlier in the priority-setting process and desired greater flexibility to collaborate with CDC. VSEs were split between these two perspectives; a few agreed that they were sufficiently involved in the process, and a few wished they could have been more involved.

Recommendations

Improve collaboration and coordination of vaccine safety information among federal agencies and more broadly

While CDC's collaboration with researchers was largely characterized as effective during the PHE, interviewees from various groups called for increased coordination between CDC and other entities. All federal agency staff and some VSD researchers and external VSEs agreed there is a need for CDC to better coordinate and streamline vaccine safety research and communications with other federal agencies, including the FDA, NIH, the Department of Defense (DoD), Department of Veterans Affairs, and Indian Health Service. A few interviewees mentioned that federal agencies appeared siloed and have limited communication despite conducting work related to that of other agencies. One VSE described how federal agencies collaborated more during the COVID-19 PHE and other PHEs; however, these enhanced collaborations were temporary, and they emphasized a need to sustain this level of collaboration over time.

Additionally, one PHO emphasized the need for CDC and federal agencies such as the Administration for Strategic Preparedness and Response to share information and updates with states immediately and specifically recommended increasing the frequency of multistate conference calls during PHEs.

Streamline processes to speed up study development and publication clearance

Most CISA researchers, some VSD researchers, and a few VSEs agreed that barriers and delays in study development and publication clearance processes need to be addressed. VSD researchers shared possible approaches for speeding up or streamlining the process, such as having multiple rounds of review happen simultaneously, only including reviewers with appropriate expertise, and better defining or limiting the scope of CDC's review process. One VSE wished CDC's cooperative agreements for publications could be eliminated. CISA researchers suggested that ISO begin consulting researchers earlier in the development of its public health priorities in order to better align study teams with reviewers; that ISO offer flexibility around proposal timing in any way possible; and that a "careful [but] not overly conservative" response to political pressures, including susceptibility to FOIA requests, would reduce operational barriers to publication.

Communications

Interview protocols for all key informant groups investigated participants' perceptions of CDC and ISO's public-facing communication strategies, public vaccine safety awareness, and public perceptions of ISO. Broadly, participants across groups praised the accuracy, credibility, and timeliness of ISO's public communications, with PHOs and HCPs yielding additional insights regarding their own efforts to make ISO's vaccine safety information more accessible. However, PHOs and HCPs also described a multitude of barriers posed by widespread misinformation and limited public awareness of ISO's vaccine safety systems. CDC-funded researchers and HCPs suggested several tactical and structural changes to improve the accessibility of and public trust in CDC's vaccine safety communications.

Successes

Transparency, timeliness, and reliability of vaccine safety information

Participants across multiple key informant groups largely perceived CDC's vaccine safety information as transparent, timely, and reliable. A few PHOs, VSEs, and HCPs noted the value of ACIP in relation to the quality of CDC's vaccine safety information, with a few VSEs and HCPs specifically describing ACIP as being transparent and responsive. All PHOs commended the speed at which CDC produced and disseminated vaccine safety information, with a few noting that CDC was successful despite the challenging circumstances of the PHE. One CISA researcher also noted that high-impact research findings were disseminated very rapidly.

Most PHOs also touched on the reliability of CDC's vaccine safety information. They described CDC as a trusted resource throughout the pandemic and noted that they encouraged the public to trust CDC's guidance as well.

Usage of accessible and tailored communication strategies

PHOs and HCPs both reported using accessible and tailored communication strategies to ensure underserved groups received vaccine safety information. For example, all PHOs explained that vaccine safety communications were translated into different languages and adapted for different reading levels. A few PHOs and HCPs also described using trusted messengers or community representatives to disseminate information to underserved populations.

Accurate representation of CDC-funded research in CDC's public-facing communications

All CISA and most VSD researchers agreed that their research was accurately represented and described in CDC's public-facing communications. One VSD researcher shared an example in which CDC staff consulted the researchers before presenting study findings to ensure they were not misinterpreting or misstating study results. Federal agency staff also reported no significant disagreements with CDC on the interpretation or reporting of vaccine safety signals.

Challenges

Limited knowledge of ACIP and vaccine safety systems

Most VSEs and HCPs agreed that the public has limited awareness or understanding of ACIP and ISO's vaccine safety systems, and this posed substantial barriers to effective vaccine safety communication. Most of the HCPs who were interviewed were all affiliated with ACIP in some capacity and noted that their colleagues, administrators, and patients generally had little or no awareness of ACIP and vaccine safety systems; therefore, they served as their workplaces' primary source of information during the PHE. One HCP described how the substantial lack of awareness in their workplace inhibited patient and clinician use of the vaccine safety systems. A PHO corroborated that they frequently needed to include an explanation about the Vaccine Adverse Event Reporting System (VAERS) in communications materials.

Misinformation and responding to public concerns

All HCPs and most PHOs cited misinformation as a pervasive barrier to effective vaccine safety communication, and they reported that CDC did not thoroughly respond to or refute instances of misinformation. HCPs unanimously stated that CDC's spokespeople and communications staff did not comprehensively address public concerns arising from misinformation, noting that CDC communications staff failed to address legitimate questions or concerns from the public possibly because the questions were regarded as unscientific or silly. Furthermore, all HCPs agreed that CDC's ineffective response to misinformation hampered their own vaccine safety communication efforts. Almost all PHOs reported that misinformation posed major communication challenges; however, several said they developed processes to address it during the PHE. These processes are described in more detail in Section D along with other successes reported by PHOs.

Recommendations

Improve accessibility and clarity of public-facing vaccine safety communications

While many interviewees commended the transparency, timeliness, and reliability of CDC ISO's vaccine safety information, some still felt there was room for improvement. All CISA and most VSD researchers suggested making communications more accessible to the public, for example, by translating research findings into plain language. Several PHOs agreed and specifically suggested that CDC communication materials be made accessible at the beginning of or early in a PHE to ensure quick dissemination to the public, rather than requiring additional time and steps to adapt language later.

All VSEs and several VSD and CISA researchers emphasized the importance of CDC effectively balancing the goals of informing the public of vaccine safety issues while still promoting public trust in vaccines. A few CISA researchers and a few VSEs felt that CDC should more clearly communicate the level of evidence or support for different vaccine safety signals. For example, they thought it would be useful for CDC to differentiate between safety signals identified in unverified VAERS reports and safety signals identified in rigorous studies, since some safety signals with little supporting evidence could be taken out of context by the public and used to draw inaccurate or incomplete conclusions.

Strengthen vaccine safety communications capacity

Interviewees from multiple groups provided suggestions for bolstering the capacity of CDC's vaccine safety communications. All HCPs advocated for more resources and funding toward communications. Most CISA researchers desired to contribute to public-facing communications about their research findings to ensure accurate presentation of data; they recommended that CDC specifically allocate funding with the purpose of involving researchers in communications development. Most HCPs strongly recommended having credentialed health professionals with neutral political stances serve as CDC's spokespeople for vaccine safety communications to increase public trust.

D. FINDINGS: DISTINCT THEMES BY GROUP

CDC VSD Sites

Vaccine Safety Datalink (VSD) is a collaborative project between CDC ISO and healthcare organizations across the United States. VSD monitors the safety of vaccines and conducts studies about rare and serious adverse events following immunization. The group of VSD researchers interviewed were leaders from seven of the 13 sites who each had extensive experience planning and executing vaccine safety studies. The group included multiple VSD site PIs or co-PIs, many of whom were physicians, epidemiologists, or biostatisticians. These researchers have published numerous studies and made recommendations to ACIP. All interviewees were a part of VSD during and after the COVID-19 PHE.

Successes

VSD researchers agreed that the infrastructure of VSD was highly effective in supporting their work during the COVID-19 PHE.

VSD infrastructure facilitated rapid and responsive vaccine safety research

As noted in theme "Effective structures and processes during the PHE" in Section C above, VSD researchers reported that the infrastructure and contract structure of VSD enabled them to rapidly respond to vaccine safety research needs during the COVID-19 PHE. While this perspective was not exclusive to VSD researchers, it is worth noting that this perspective was unanimous among interviewed VSD researchers, several of whom shared additional details on the topic. One researcher mentioned specifically that the umbrella contract structure of VSD eliminated some of the bureaucratic hurdles that can hinder collaboration common in other types of contracts. Another researcher noted that their team was able to plan for COVID-19 vaccine safety research well in advance; this enabled them to begin studies as soon as vaccines were authorized. They added that key research elements, such as necessary data use agreements, project management processes, and communications streams, were all already in place.

Challenges

VSD researchers described confusion regarding communication responsibilities as being a challenge during the PHE.

Unclear who was responsible for communicating vaccine safety findings

Some VSD researchers felt they did not receive clarity regarding who was responsible for sharing findings from VSD studies with the public. Specifically, a few researchers described feeling unsure as to who was ultimately responsible for communicating vaccine safety findings—CDC ISO, CDC staff from other departments, or the VSD researchers themselves. One or two interviewees noted that VSD researchers do not typically have expertise in research communications and would require additional support if they were to play a larger role in sharing study findings.

Recommendations

VSD researchers provided several suggestions for improving vaccine safety communications.

Better support and coordination for vaccine safety communications

Although multiple key informant groups called for improved vaccine safety communications, VSD researchers shared several distinct recommendations for these communications. A few VSD researchers felt it would be valuable to adapt their study findings for communication formats besides academic journals, such as news articles and social media posts. One researcher also felt it would be valuable to distribute educational flyers or videos about their studies with participating health systems that contribute data to VSD. Several researchers who provided these recommendations noted that they would need additional support and more communications expertise to adapt study findings for communications that target various audiences. Lastly, a few researchers recommended that CDC regularly update the VSD website to ensure information about VSD and its research processes remain current and are easy to find.

CDC-Funded Researchers: CISA

The group of CISA researchers interviewed was made up of five leaders from five of eight medical research centers involved in CISA nationwide, with decades of collective experience planning and executing CISA research and clinical consultation tasks. This group included multiple CISA site PIs, medical professionals with extensive backgrounds in several specializations, and authors and leads of numerous vaccine safety studies and clinical trials. All interviewees had experience working on CISA efforts before, during, and after the PHE.

Successes

CISA researchers spoke at length about the effectiveness of ISO's leadership, infrastructure, and resource allocation during the PHE. These successes are discussed in "Successes" in Section C above.

Challenges

CISA researchers had unique concerns about their limited ability to contribute to public health communications, the level of public awareness of CISA's activities and publications, and the recent staff turnover at ISO.

Division between researchers and public-health communications may limit impact of research

Most CISA researchers described how the division between research and public-health communications functions within ISO limited the potential impact of their research and expertise on public awareness and vaccine safety. Several pointed out that CISA researchers, with their unique combination of clinical experience and specialized vaccine safety research knowledge, could provide valuable consultation on communications materials and talking points for doctors and PHOs, but the current structure of CISA restricts them from contributing to many public-health communications efforts.

Concerns about readiness after turnover at ISO

Most CISA researchers expressed concerns about the long-term readiness and capacity of ISO's staff, particularly after a period of significant turnover following the PHE. One CISA researcher also pointed out that ISO's interdepartment rotation program reduces each department's efficiency by temporarily depriving teams of the "institutional awareness" of experienced staff.

Although they generally spoke highly of the communication, leadership, and expertise of the ISO leaders in place during the PHE, these researchers spoke at length about the unique skill set needed for ISO to function well. They mentioned strong leadership, communication skills, flexibility, and the ability to navigate bureaucracy as vital characteristics for ISO staff. To these points, researchers described a great loss of institutional knowledge at ISO due to turnover that occurred between the PHE and the present day, which has reportedly impacted ISO's ability to navigate the overlapping bureaucratic structures of CDC, state public health systems, and academia.

Rigidity of ISO processes

Most CISA researchers noted there were challenges with rigidity and inefficiency in ISO's organizational structure, highlighting the restrictive timelines of ISO research grant applications and a restrictive adherence to CDC and ACIP public health priorities during study selection. A few researchers specifically expressed concerns about the current ISO management and communications teams being restricted by the priorities of CDC leadership, positing that this hampers ISO's capacity to communicate effectively rather than "toeing the line" and worrying about "saying things the right way." Researchers described how these tendencies can limit research teams' ability to work flexibly and independently, though CISA researchers did not share VSD researchers' concerns about direct ISO influence on research products and spoke highly of ISO's accurate portrayals of their research in communication products.

A few CISA researchers also mentioned they had greater clinical consultation capacity than was utilized during the PHE, and that ISO restricted the number of cases they were referred to avoid overwhelming CISA staff. Notably, this description stands in contrast to the perceptions shared by most VSEs, who perceived that CISA lacked the infrastructure to keep up with incoming adverse event reports during the PHE.

Awareness of CISA as a body is low, hampering impact of research results

Although they spoke highly of the short-term funding allocated during the pandemic (discussed in Section C), several CISA researchers expressed concern about the resources allocated to driving awareness and scaling of CISA research on an ongoing basis. Regarding ISO funding and

APPENDIX C

programmatic support, they described the treatment of CISA as a "little sibling" of VAERS and VSD, calling for more egalitarian support for CISA and better integration between the three systems. They described how limited public awareness of CISA reduces the number of HCPs and members of the public who seek out its research products and limits its potential to improve vaccine confidence through research dissemination.

Recommendations

CISA researchers included some basic suggestions for improvement in their descriptions of the challenges described above. They also offered recommendations for better integrating research teams into ISO's research priority-setting process.

Desire for researchers to be more involved in study or grant priority setting

Almost all CISA researchers described how, in earlier iterations of the CISA program years before the PHE, ISO's process for designating research priorities was more researcher-driven. However, in more recent years, they mentioned that priorities were mostly discussed internally within CDC, with the process being a "black box" from the researcher's perspective. Several researchers mentioned that they did approve of CDC's research priorities and that they were consulted to some extent in recent years, but others asked to be more included. They proposed a start-of-year meeting between ISO and its funded researchers to gauge priorities among the research community, and in one case called passionately for academics to be more involved in the development of project best practices and funding priorities, referring to the strict imposition of a "top-down CDC way" in recent years. As mentioned in Section C, VSD researchers described a much more positive account of their own involvement in priority setting.

Healthcare Professionals

Interviewed HCPs ($n=4$) worked in a variety of settings, including clinical, academic, and nonprofit institutions. It is important to note that all interviewed HCPs were affiliated with ACIP, and not all were practicing clinicians during the COVID-19 PHE; as such, they sometimes referred to the experiences or perspectives of colleagues who were practicing and had direct interactions with patients during that time. Interviews with HCPs focused on understanding their perceptions of and experiences with the four vaccine safety systems, as well as professional- and public-facing vaccine safety communications.

Successes

HCPs described successes in using targeted approaches to communicate vaccine safety information to underserved patient populations.

Trusted community representatives helped with communicating vaccine safety information to patients from underserved groups

Half the HCPs noted that using trusted community messengers was an effective approach for communicating vaccine safety information to patients from underserved groups. For example, they described having female and Black clinicians share information with pregnant and Black patients, respectively. Half the HCPs also mentioned that effectively communicating with underserved patients was especially important since they had less access to information and more often expressed vaccine-related concerns.

Challenges

As mentioned previously in the discussion of the "Communications" theme in Section C, most challenges reported by HCPs were tied to vaccine safety communications.

Clinicians, health administrators, and patients had limited awareness of ACIP and vaccine safety systems

Most HCPs reported that their colleagues, institution's leaders, and patients had limited or no awareness of ACIP or the vaccine safety systems during the COVID-19 PHE. Some HCPs indicated that if they had not mentioned ACIP or the vaccine safety systems at their workplaces, their colleagues, leaders, and patients would likely not have been informed about these topics. However, they noted that some patients may have seen related information on social media.

Lack of refutations to misinformation hindered the effectiveness of communications

All HCPs expressed that CDC did not effectively refute misinformation about vaccine safety, nor did they thoroughly address public concerns regarding vaccines during the COVID-19 PHE. They described CDC's communication approaches as rigid and using technical jargon, which ultimately failed to address questions from the public that were perceived as silly or unscientific.

Recommendations

To overcome the challenges described above, HCPs recommended that CDC enhance the capacity and credibility of their communication efforts.

Increase funding for vaccine safety systems education and communications

All HCPs called for significant increases in the amount of funding allocated to CDC's vaccine safety communications, as well as more public-facing vaccine safety education initiatives and enhancements to CDC's communication infrastructure and processes.

Utilize a credentialed, unbiased professional as vaccine safety spokesperson

Most HCPs recommended that CDC appoint a credentialed health professional who is unbiased and not politically driven to be a vaccine safety spokesperson to communicate information externally. HCPs indicated that designating a spokesperson who has these qualities is crucial for building public trust in vaccines and improving the coordination of vaccine safety information.

Vaccine Safety Experts

VSEs ($n=6$) were primarily external researchers focused on vaccine safety. Interviews with VSEs aimed to understand their experiences using the four vaccine safety systems, perceptions regarding data transparency, and experiences with publishing vaccine safety research.

Successes

Most successes reported by VSEs pertained to ACIP's transparency during public-facing meetings and specific components or attributes of the four vaccine safety systems.

Data transparency was valuable in ACIP meetings

Half the VSEs described the value of ACIP openly sharing vaccine safety information during their public-facing meetings throughout the COVID-19

PHE. A few VSEs mentioned they felt it was ACIP's "duty" or "role" to be transparent with the public. One VSE mentioned that ACIP was also responsive to safety concerns brought forward by clinicians during their meetings.

Vaccine safety systems' benefits: CISA's case consults, VAERS' rapid surveillance methods, V-safe's text capabilities, VSD's scientific rigor

Most VSEs reported that CISA's case consultations were valuable. Specifically, they noted that CISA's clinician consultants efficiently provided individual-level vaccine safety recommendations, and they also liked CISA's structure, which is composed of clinicians proactively working together to address adverse vaccine events. Most VSEs mentioned that VSD's level of scientific rigor, active surveillance methods, and wide scope and reach were highly valuable for research. Half the VSEs reported that VAERS' rapid surveillance methods were efficient for quick signal detection and data collection and analysis. Additionally, half the VSEs liked V-safe's text message capabilities; one VSE described how this modality of communication conveyed to the public that researchers were interested in addressing and responding to their adverse events.

Challenges

Challenges reported by VSEs pertained to pitfalls or limitations of the four vaccine safety systems, as well as barriers associated with prioritizing and publishing vaccine safety research.

Vaccine safety systems' limitations: VAERS data can be misused, CISA's case consults were underutilized, V-safe has limited infrastructure, VSD has limited data

All VSEs reported that VAERS data were misused or misinterpreted and had limited scientific rigor due to its passive surveillance methods. They discussed specific limitations of VAERS, including that its data was underreported, biased, and incomplete due to self-reporting, and that it lacked clear case definitions. Most VSEs perceived that CISA is significantly underfunded, underused, and has insufficient infrastructure to follow up on all reported adverse events. Half the VSEs also mentioned that V-safe lacked sufficient infrastructure to support adverse event follow-up, similar to CISA. They noted that the initial intention of V-safe's text messaging service was to respond to all individuals who reported adverse events; however, they felt that V-safe's staff quickly became overwhelmed by the number of messages and were unable to respond to them. Finally, most

VSEs noted limitations of VSD's structure; these included observations that VSD's database did not always have sufficient data to stratify adverse events by subpopulations (e.g., different age groups) and VSD's data was more difficult to access than VAERS.

Cooperative agreements and prioritization of leaders' research interests

Some VSEs described challenges associated with prioritizing and publishing or sharing vaccine safety research. Two VSEs reported each of the following challenges: delays in publishing research due to CDC cooperative agreements that required a CDC employee to coauthor manuscripts; CDC ISO's reluctance to pursue or publish research that does not align with leaders' interests or may be deemed as controversial; and insufficient collaboration between CDC ISO, other federal agencies, and external vaccine researchers and institutions.

Recommendations

Overarching recommendations from VSEs pertained to increasing the structural capacity, funding, and resources put toward vaccine safety systems, both during and outside of PHE contexts.

More funding for vaccine safety system infrastructure, particularly supporting follow-up to reported adverse events

All VSEs called for more sustained funding and resources put toward vaccine safety systems. They indicated that the challenges encountered during the COVID-19 PHE would repeat in the future if more funding and resources are not allocated to these systems. Most VSEs specifically recommended that additional support be put toward reported adverse event follow-up efforts to address the challenges described above.

Sustained interagency and external collaborations

Half the VSEs called for sustained collaborations among federal agencies as well as with external institutions (e.g., academic institutions and international organizations). They noted that CDC ISO is only one "player" in the vaccine safety space, and that CDC ISO would benefit from stronger partnerships with the FDA, NIH, DoD, and the Veterans Health Administration.

Furthermore, some VSEs recommended that CDC ISO more proactively work with and listen to vaccine safety researchers employed at academic institutions and other organizations (e.g., the WHO).

State and Local Public Health Officials

State and local PHOs ($n=5$) shared successes, challenges, and recommendations regarding vaccine safety information sources and described communication strategies for disseminating vaccine safety information to the public. Due to the small sample size, we did not differentiate findings by state and local perspectives.

Successes

PHOs found value in collaborative partnerships and continued to disseminate accurate and reliable sources of information to the public despite misinformation challenges.

Positive, collaborative relationship between state and local health departments and other partners

Sustaining partnerships was integral for mobilizing and disseminating a consistent message within states regarding COVID-19 and vaccine safety. Most PHOs described having positive, collaborative relationships within their respective state and local health departments and with hospital systems, healthcare providers, elected officials, law enforcement and emergency services, and community partners. For example, one PHO described their health department as a "regional hub" for supporting various entities to effectively guide the public through the PHE.

Development of communication strategies to address the public's vaccine safety concerns and mitigate the spread of misinformation

Most PHOs recognized there were sources of misinformation that could influence vaccine safety communication efforts. Some PHOs discussed the importance of developing processes for acknowledging and addressing public concerns, even if they were unfounded or "silly," and they described a few strategies they used to get ahead of the spread of misinformation. One PHO's health department reported success using a vaccine safety hotline to address the public's questions and concerns and hiding any posts or comments that were spreading misinformation on the health department's social media platforms. Another PHO encouraged frontline staff at vaccine clinics to leverage one-on-one conversations with patients as an opportunity to connect and encourage vaccine trust.

Challenges

PHOs experienced challenges navigating misinformation and constant changes to public health and vaccine safety guidance.

Misinformation was a persistent public-health and vaccine-safety communication issue

Many PHOs described misinformation as a primary contributing factor to vaccine hesitancy and distrust. Some PHOs described how conflicting public health guidance provided early in the COVID-19 PHE fueled public confusion and concern; for example, rapidly changing guidance regarding masks was viewed as unclear. One PHO attributed vaccine distrust and confusion to publicizing the vaccine manufacturing process without providing adequate context for the years of research and testing that contributed to the vaccine's development. Nearly all PHOs mentioned that unverified VAERS reports often fueled public misinformation.

CDC's public health and vaccine safety information was unclear and delayed at times

All PHOs understood that COVID-19 and vaccine safety information rapidly changed as research evolved during the PHE; however, many PHOs struggled to identify guidance updates. Some PHOs described CDC's website as a "tangled web" that can be challenging to navigate even for the most experienced individuals. Another PHO expressed frustration with learning information at the same time as the public and feeling unprepared to address the public's questions without adequate notice of updated guidance.

Recommendations

PHOs suggested improvements on how to provide clear and complete public health and vaccine safety information and minimize the potential for misinformation to erode public trust in the process.

Acknowledge guidance will change as new data emerges

Although all PHOs found it challenging to keep up with rapidly changing guidance, they appreciated CDC's transparency in informing the public as new data emerged. A few PHOs encouraged CDC to consider acknowledging unknown circumstances at the onset of PHEs to minimize confusion or skepticism when guidance changes.

Clearly identify changes to vaccine safety guidance

Most PHOs recommended that when changing prior or existing guidance, CDC should clearly highlight the changes to make it easier for people to identify new or updated information. They also recommended that communications be dated and time-stamped and include a summary of what changes were made and why so that PHOs can efficiently identify and then disseminate updated guidance to the public.

Develop a provider-facing and public-facing system for VAERS reports

Some PHOs recommended CDC develop a provider-facing and public-facing system for VAERS reports. PHOs appreciated having VAERS reports as a reference when talking to patients who experienced an adverse event, but PHOs encouraged CDC to consider a public-facing system that contextualizes the adverse events to help the public better understand vaccine risk and the role of reporting systems as a vaccine safety tool.

E. CONCLUSIONS

This qualitative study assessed key informants' views regarding CDC ISO's systems, methods, and processes pertaining to COVID-19 vaccine safety during the U.S. COVID-19 PHE. Key informants, who included federal agency staff, CDC-funded researchers, HCPs, outside VSEs, and state and local PHOs, shared perspectives reflecting an array of professional disciplines integral to vaccine safety and communications during the PHE.

Study Limitations

Although this study yielded important insights regarding CDC ISO and vaccine safety efforts, it had a low sample size, with $n \leq 7$ participants from each key informant group. The perspectives expressed by participants in this study are not necessarily generalizable to other researchers, HCPs, VSEs, or PHOs. Westat's pool of participants was derived essentially from a convenience sample, as opposed to a randomly drawn sample from the full population of each key informant group. While this approach was appropriate for the Committee's aims and the available time and resources for conducting the study, there are unavoidable selection and sampling biases inherent in this approach. For example, the population of HCPs during the PHE is much greater than Westat or NASEM could identify, sample, and conduct outreach to for this study. However, for VSD sites, we were able to start with a complete population and reach a much larger proportion of sites.

Numerous study participants were connected with ACIP in some capacity and/or shared perspectives from roles other than those tied to their key informant group (or those that occurred outside the COVID-19

APPENDIX C

PHE). Thus, some participants' responses were not necessarily representative of non-ACIP-affiliated professionals and/or could have been affected by recall bias. Some participants referenced their colleagues' or patients' perspectives in response to certain questions for which they had limited knowledge.

Most importantly, Westat was unable to interview individuals who were employed at CDC during the COVID-19 PHE, per direction from CDC ISO leadership. As such, perspectives from this critical key informant group were missing from our analysis. Additionally, only a very limited pool of other federal staff working with ISO were able to be identified.

Other limitations of this study were tied to interview durations, participants' unwillingness or inability to answer certain questions, and the potential for additional biases in the small-group interviews. Regarding interview durations, Westat was not always able to ask all questions on the interview guides if participants provided extensive details or wanted to focus on specific topics. Additionally, some questions were deemed not applicable to certain participants due to their lack of personal experience or perspectives regarding those topics. Participants may have also limited their responses to certain questions due to concerns regarding political sensitivities associated with the topic of vaccine safety. In the handful of small-group interviews consisting of two participants, participants' responses could have been influenced by peer responses and social desirability biases.

Finally, this study primarily focused on processes during the PHE. As a result, the findings may not reflect current CDC policies and procedures.

Overarching Findings

Despite the limitations discussed above, the results of this study can be used to provide insight into the strengths and limitations of the systems and processes in place during the PHE and the array of challenges faced by these key informant groups, as well as to identify potential improvements for further examination and areas for additional research and evaluation.

Successes and Challenges

Overall, key informants reported that CDC ISO's COVID-19 vaccine safety efforts were strong; however, they noted substantial challenges and presented recommendations to enhance CDC ISO's efforts moving forward. With regards to infrastructure, resources, and processes, key informants from most groups commended the existing structures of the four vaccine safety systems (CISA, VAERS, VSD, and V-safe), enhanced processes during the PHE, and increased resources and funding during the PHE. They emphasized that these fundamental operational components, combined with CDC ISO's effective leadership, enabled rapid COVID-19 vaccine safety research and emergency response efforts. However, they conveyed that vaccine safety structures, resources, and processes were still insufficient, and CDC ISO's COVID-19 response would have been stronger with additional funding and staff, and a more robust infrastructure.

Key informants' perspectives regarding CDC ISO's coordination and collaboration with other agencies and researchers during the COVID-19 PHE were largely positive. CDC-funded researchers and VSEs shared contrasting views regarding their level of involvement and ability to provide input into CDC ISO's vaccine safety research, especially priority setting. Some CDC- funded researchers and VSEs expressed concerns with CDC's research clearance and publishing procedures, which created delays and reduced their scientific independence.

Regarding communications, key informants from multiple groups perceived CDC's and ACIP's vaccine safety information as transparent, timely, and trustworthy. CDC-funded researchers largely felt that their findings were accurately represented in CDC's public-facing communications. HCPs and PHOs described successes in adapting CDC's vaccine safety communications for various audiences. However, key informants across multiple groups discussed pervasive challenges with COVID-19 and vaccine-related misinformation, and they indicated that CDC did not thoroughly address public concerns or debunk misinformation. They also noted that the public, other HCPs, and health administrators have limited or no understanding of ACIP and the four vaccine safety systems, which posed substantial barriers to effective communication during the PHE.

Recommendations

As discussed throughout this report, key informants presented recommendations to address vaccine safety process and communication challenges encountered during the COVID-19 PHE. Additionally, their recommendations aimed to strengthen future PHE preparedness and response efforts.

Key informants noted that it is of the utmost importance to continue building CDC ISO's vaccine safety systems and infrastructure. They recommended increasing and sustaining the amount of funding and resources allocated toward the four vaccine safety systems over the long term. Key informants also called for a more proactive approach to monitoring and addressing potential vaccine safety issues. Additionally, they recommended that CDC ISO increase and sustain their collaborations with other federal agencies and external researchers/entities outside of PHE contexts to ensure proactiveness and preparedness. Several

APPENDIX C

CDC-funded researchers and VSEs described a need to alleviate barriers with CDC's research clearance and publication processes to reduce delays and promote scientific independence.

To strengthen public awareness of and trust in vaccine safety efforts, key informants recommended that more funding should be allocated to CDC's vaccine safety communications, and that CDC's vaccine safety information should be shared externally by an unbiased spokesperson who is credentialed in the health sciences. Lastly, key informants recommended that CDC create more accessible vaccine safety information materials and more clearly communicate the level of evidence for different safety signals to strengthen the public's trust in vaccines.

Areas Warranting Further Examination

The perspectives and experiences of these key informants suggest additional examination of issues and processes may be beneficial to CDC ISO's long-term improvement efforts. Regarding the infrastructure, systems, and resources for vaccine safety research and communication, a full understanding of the scope and impact of any resource increases occurring during the PHE is needed and warrants further study. Additionally, further study is necessary to develop more detailed recommendations regarding the appropriate amount of resources, staff, and funding that should be allocated to specific vaccine safety systems, processes, and communications.

Information on program specific resource changes and the inclusion of agency staff perspectives would both benefit that examination.

Interviews with VSD and CISA researchers also suggest that structural and process differences in these two systems may be affecting their views of the effectiveness of collaboration. As these systems have different objectives, their processes are necessarily different; however, the identification of system-specific improvements requires more in-depth study. Similarly, there may be value in deeper examination of methods for ensuring engagement and collaboration with external VSEs and researchers. The small pool of external VSEs included in this study offered insights on several vaccine safety systems that other key informants largely did not raise.

Recommendations for process improvements across all four vaccine safety systems requires additional input and further study.

Moreover, further examination of publication clearance challenges and timeliness would be beneficial to more clearly identify and evaluate process improvements. Case studies examining the factors influencing the publication process for a sample of papers could help to facilitate the development of specific recommendations.

Lastly, a more targeted study of communication specialists within CDC, other agencies, and at the state and local level (including Tribal Health Service Areas) would offer valuable insights regarding vaccine safety communication challenges and improvements. This study largely included researchers and HCPs. To further investigate effective methods for tailoring vaccine safety communications for various audiences (researchers, HCPs, and the public) and to ensure transparency and understanding of research on safety signals, insights from communication specialists in this area are needed.

APPENDIX A. INTERVIEW GUIDES

Introductory Script for All Interviews

Thanks very much for agreeing to speak with us. My name is (if applicable: and I'm here with .) We're from Westat, a health and social policy research organization. In early 2024, the Centers for Disease Control and Prevention Immunization Safety Office (CDC ISO) asked the National Academies of Sciences, Engineering, and Medicine (NASEM) to evaluate CDC ISO's systems, methods, and processes for monitoring COVID-19 vaccine safety during the COVID-19 public health emergency. We have been funded by the NASEM to conduct confidential interviews and focus groups as part of that consensus study.

We're conducting this interview with you today as part of this evaluation. The goal of this discussion is to better understand key stakeholders' perspectives regarding CDC ISO's vaccine safety processes, priorities, communications, and collaborations during the COVID-19 emergency. We're speaking with individuals from numerous key informant groups, including CDC staff, ISO contractors, staff from other federal, state, and local health agencies, healthcare professionals, and other vaccine researchers. Ultimately, insights shared through these interviews and focus groups will be used to develop recommendations for sustaining, maintaining, and strengthening CDC ISO's vaccine safety monitoring systems and communications.

We have a series of questions to guide our discussion. You may not know the answer to every question, and there are no right or wrong answers. We are interested in your individual perspective. Your participation in this [interview/focus group] is voluntary. If there are any questions that you don't feel knowledgeable about or don't feel comfortable answering, please let us know, and we will move on.

[Only if focus group/multi-person interview]: We will also be using a tool called a Mural Board that allows you to anonymously comment and respond to the discussion.

You should have received a copy of the consent form via email prior to this meeting. It explains much of the information I just reviewed, including why we are conducting this [interview/focus group].

[Only if focus group]: As we noted there, because this is a focus group, you all are of course aware of each other's participation and will have knowledge of each of your perspectives. We ask all of you to respect the privacy of each other and not disclose other participants' feedback.

Information gathered during our [interview/focus group] will be used in combination with other interviews and focus groups in a summary report which will be available on NASEM's website. None of the information you share with us today will be attributed to you personally in any way. We are interviewing many people for this study, and we will paraphrase, rather than direct quote, participants. Agency and organization names will be mentioned, but again, no individuals will be directly identified. We'll be taking notes during our discussion, and if [you/everyone] agrees, we will record this discussion as a backup to those notes.

Please note: the recording, transcript, and notes from our discussion will be stored on Westat's secure server and will only be accessible to the Westat staff working on this study. Any sensitive material, including personally identifiable information (PII), will be redacted from transcripts and notes. Recordings will be deleted upon review and redaction of PII from transcripts and notes. All other data, such as transcripts and analytic files, will be destroyed after the overall study is completed and published.

Since this is a videoconference, we strongly encourage you to participate in a private setting away from others. Also, while we are employing all appropriate security measures during this virtual interview, it is important that you know that no system such as Zoom is 100 percent secure.

1. Do you have any questions?
2. Do you agree to proceed with our interview or not?
3. Do you agree to have this conversation recorded or not?

[Note to researchers: If the key informant does not give permission to record, proceed with the interview. In this case, it is essential that the non-interviewing researcher(s) on the team take extensive notes, capturing as much detail as possible.]

Federal Government Staff Guide

Interviewee's Role

I'd like to start by learning about your work and area of expertise and focus. This is to help us interpret your responses and analyze them. We will not directly quote you or refer to your position directly in our summary report.

1. What is your area of expertise/position?
2. What was your role or focus during the COVID-19 emergency?

Resource Allocation

We'd like to learn about your experiences during the COVID-19 emergency starting in March 2020 through May 2023. Let's start by talking about vaccine safety resource allocation.

3. [P] Thinking back to the time of the COVID-19 emergency, how did resourcing for vaccine safety evaluation, assessment and research change?
4. Was additional funding made available to your agency? What was the additional funding used for? What was impact (positive/negative)?
5. [P] Were additional staff hired/brought in to support vaccine safety evaluation, assessment and research? What were their roles?
6. [P] What was the impact of these changes?
7. [P] Have programmatic resourcing increases (new efforts, new staff, funding streams) targeted to Covid vaccine safety been retained post COVID-19 emergency? If so, in what areas/what ways?

Vaccine Safety Evaluation, Assessment and Research Priorities

8. How do you/ does your organization set priorities for vaccine safety evaluation, assessment and research? How does that align with CDC's priorities?
   a. How effective is that process? Did it change during the COVID-19 emergency, and if so, how?
9. [P] How do you/ does your organization engage with CDC ISO in setting priorities for vaccine safety evaluation, assessment and research?
   a. [P] Is this engagement sufficient? How can vaccine safety evaluation, assessment and research collaborations with CDC ISO be improved?

10. How do the evaluation, assessment and research priorities differ between you/your organization (or office) and CDC ISO?
    a. How did that impact (benefit or hinder) your mission or overall vaccine safety research?

Coordination in Federal Vaccine Safety Efforts

Our next several questions pertain to coordination efforts between numerous organizations, systems, and processes that contribute to vaccine safety.

11. [P] From your perspective, how robust and effectively coordinated are vaccine safety efforts within the federal government?
12. Are coordination mechanisms adequate to prevent unnecessary duplication of effort or to ensure optimal vaccine safety and community?
    a. If there are coordination gaps, what are they and what are their impacts?
    b. How could these coordination gaps be addressed?
13. [P] How could federal vaccine safety efforts be improved overall?

Public Communication

Lastly, we'd like to discuss efforts pertaining to vaccine safety communication.

14. What was your agency's process for determining vaccine communications content/messages?
15. [P] How was this process coordinated within your agency and with CDC's ISO and what other agencies or stakeholders were involved?
16. [P] Did vaccine safety communications differ in terms of content or prioritization between your agency and CDC ISO?
17. [P] During the COVID-19 emergency, what formal guidance or criteria, if any, was provided for communications about potential vaccine safety issues?
    a. Were there competing organizational perspectives on the right approach for communicating potential safety issues?
    b. If so, how were these adjudicated?
    c. Can you think of a time when a safety issue message was enhanced or softened as it went through the adjudication process?
18. [P] If your office or agency put out vaccine safety information, how did that information or guidance change over time during and after the COVID-19 emergency?

Those are all the questions I have for you today. Is there anything else you'd like to share regarding your experiences during the COVID-19 emergency?

Thank you so much for taking the time to share your experiences and feedback. This concludes our discussion. Have a great rest of your day!

ISO Funded Researchers - VSD

Interviewee's Role

I'd like to start by learning about your role within VSD and your area of expertise or focus. This is to help us interpret your responses and analyze them. We will not be directly citing or referring to your position in our summary report.

1. What is your role or area of expertise (what are your current responsibilities)?
2. Was your role during the COVID-19 emergency different from what you had been doing prior to the COVID-19 emergency?

Vaccine Safety Evaluation, Assessment and Research Priorities and Independence

First, we'd like to learn about how vaccine safety research and evaluation priorities are determined within the VSD project.

3. What is the process for setting vaccine safety research and evaluation priorities within VSD and within your site?
   a. [P] What works well in this process and what is challenging?
   b. How could this be improved?
4. [P] Did the process for setting priorities change during the COVID-19 emergency? If so, how?
5. Did you feel that you had input into CDC ISO's overall process of setting research priorities around vaccine safety assessment and communications? Why or why not?

Relationship with CDC

Now, we'd like to learn about your experiences during the COVID-19 emergency starting in March 2020 through May 2023. Let's start by talking about your relationship with CDC.

APPENDIX C

6. [P] In what ways did your relationship with CDC change during the transition from non- emergency or routine vaccination safety assessment, evaluation and research to the COVID-19 public health emergency response?
   a. [P] What worked well? What were the challenges?
   b. Were there ways in which your relationship with CDC could have been improved?
7. [P] Please describe any changes made during the COVID-19 emergency you feel had an impact on your work. These could be evaluation, assessment or research-related changes or administrative or procedural changes.
8. Were there challenges due to these changes? How did they help or improve your work?
9. What other improvements or changes were needed?
10. Are there changes that you think should or should not have remained in place when transitioning back to non-emergency operations?
11. How does your experience working with ISO compare with your experience working with other research funding sources, including industry (note to interviewer – this often is tied more to contract type and should potentially be asked about)?
    a. In what ways is it similar? How is it different?
    b. In terms of independence? Ease of collaboration? Publishing? Speed and ease of contracting, other mechanisms?
12. [P] How effective was the leadership provided by ISO during the pandemic?
13. Were there any challenges you or your organization encountered with the CDC contracting process? How is it now?
    a. How can the contracting process be improved, if at all?
14. [P] Have you ever experienced a situation in which there was disagreement between you or your team and ISO on the seriousness of a vaccine safety or how to respond to a vaccine safety signal (timeliness of reporting, etc.)?
    a. What happened as a result of the disagreement or how was the disagreement resolved?
    b. Did this situation occur during the COVID-19 emergency? Does being in an emergency response situation change the process for addressing situations like this?
    c. What changes or improvements could be made to resolve these situations?

Communication and Public Perception

Next, we'd like to discuss how CDC communicated the results of vaccine safety evaluation, assessment and research to the public.

15. [P] How effectively do you think CDC communicates research findings to healthcare professionals and the public, especially individuals from marginalized groups?
    a. Did you feel that your work was sufficiently shared/distributed?
16. [P] During the COVID-19 emergency (or at any other time), did you experience a time in which you were surprised by or disagreed with how a CDC communication described VSD research? Can you describe this situation?
17. [P] What changes could be made to improve CDC's process for communicating findings from VSD research?

General Experience During Public Health Emergency and Suggestions for Improvement

The last few questions are about your general experiences during the COVID-19 emergency and how you feel systems, processes, research, and communication could be improved.

18. [P] What would you recommend to improve CDC's safety monitoring efforts going forward (aside from additional funding)?
19. [P] How can CDC vaccine safety researchers improve public communications pertaining to vaccine safety research?
20. What was your biggest accomplishment during the COVID-19 emergency and what made it successful?
21. [If needed] What was your biggest disappointment during the COVID-19 emergency?

Those are all of the questions I have for you today. Is there anything else you'd like to share regarding your experiences during the COVID-19 emergency?

Thank you so much for taking the time to share your experiences and feedback.

APPENDIX C   163

ISO Funded Researchers - CISA

Interviewee's Role

I'd like to start by learning about your role and area of expertise and focus. This is to help us interpret your responses and analyze them. We will not be directly citing or referring to your position in our summary report.

1. What is your role/area of expertise (what are your current responsibilities)?
2. Was your role during the COVID-19 emergency the same as prior to the COVID-19 emergency or did you assume a new role or position during the COVID-19 emergency? What office were you in?

Vaccine Safety Evaluation, Assessment and Research Priorities and Independence

First, we'd like to learn about how vaccine safety research and evaluation priorities are determined within [CISA].

3. How do you set your vaccine safety research and evaluation priorities or how are they set within CISA?
   a. [P] What works well in this process and what is challenging? How could this be improved?
4. [P] Did the process for setting priorities change during the COVID-19 emergency? If so, how?
5. Did you feel that your work/results (or input on priorities) were appropriately incorporated in CDC ISO's overall process of vaccine safety assessment and communications? Why or why not?
6. Did you feel that your work was sufficiently shared/distributed?

Relationship with CDC

Now, we'd like to learn about your experiences during the COVID-19 emergency starting in March 2020 through May 2023. Let's start by talking about your relationship with CDC.

7. [P] In what ways did your relationship with CDC change during the transition from non- emergency/routine vaccination safety assessment, evaluation and research to the COVID-19 public health emergency response period of time (3/2020 to 5/2023)?

How did your safety assessment, evaluation, research and work change?
a. [P] What worked well? What were the challenges?
b. How could your relationship with CDC have been improved?
8. [P] Please describe any evaluation, assessment or research-related or administrative or procedural changes made during the COVID-19 emergency you feel had an impact on your work.
a. Were there challenges due to these changes? How did they help or improve your work?
b. What other improvements or changes were needed?
c. Are there changes that you think should or should not have remained in place when transitioning back to non-emergency operations?
9. How does your experience working with ISO compare with your experience working with other research funding sources, including industry (note to interviewer – this often is tied more to contract type and should potentially be asked about)?
a. In what ways is it similar? How is it different?
b. In terms of independence? Ease of collaboration? Publishing? Speed and ease of contracting, other mechanisms?
10. [P] Describe the quality or effectiveness (clarity) of leadership provided by CDC during the pandemic? Were there any challenges you encountered with the CDC contracting process? How is it now?
a. How can the contracting process be improved, if at all?
11. [P] Have you ever experienced a situation in which there was disagreement between you/your team and CDC on the seriousness and response to a vaccine safety signal (timeliness of reporting, etc.)?
a. What happened as a result of the disagreement or how was the disagreement resolved?
b. Did this situation occur during the COVID-19 emergency? Does being in an emergency response situation change the process for addressing situations like this?
c. What changes or improvements could be made to resolve these situations?

Communication and Public Perception

Next, we'd like to discuss how CDC communicated the results of vaccine safety evaluation, assessment and research to the public.

12. [P] How effectively do you think CDC communicates research

APPENDIX C

findings to healthcare professionals and the public, especially individuals from marginalized groups?
13. [P] During the COVID-19 emergency (or at any time alternatively), did you experience a time in which you were surprised by or disagreed with how a CDC communication described CISA research? Can you describe this situation?
14. [P] What changes could be made to improve CDC's process for communicating findings from CISA research?

General Experience During Public Health Emergency and Suggestions for Improvement

The last few questions pertain to your general experiences during the COVID-19 emergency and how you feel systems, processes, research, and communication could be improved.

15. What was your biggest accomplishment during the COVID-19 emergency and what made it successful?
16. [If needed] What was your biggest disappointment during the COVID-19 emergency?
17. [P] What would you recommend to improve CDC's safety monitoring efforts going forward (aside from additional funding)?
18. [P] How can CDC vaccine safety researchers improve public communications pertaining to vaccine safety research?

Those are all of the questions I have for you today. Is there anything else you'd like to share regarding your experiences during the COVID-19 emergency?

Thank you so much for taking the time to share your experiences and feedback.

Healthcare Professionals

Interviewee's Role

I'd like to start with brief introductions.

1. What is your area of expertise/profession? [Note: If they mentioned this in the survey, consider rephrasing to "You mentioned your area of focus is X.. Is there anything else you'd like to share about your profession or areas of expertise?"
2. What was your role or focus during the COVID-19 emergency (from March 2020 through May 2023)?

Vaccine Safety Systems

Next, we'd like to learn about your experiences as a healthcare professional during the COVID-19 emergency, starting in March 2020 through May 2023. Let's start by talking about your familiarity and experience with the CDC ISO's vaccine safety systems. [May require providing some brief info on CDC ISO role vs FDA.]

3. [P] [If they did not indicate this in the survey] Which of the following vaccine safety reporting systems are you aware of: V-safe, VAERS, VSD, or CISA?
4. [P] [If aware of V-safe] How were patients encouraged to use V-safe to report vaccine side effects by either you or your colleagues in your practice during the COVID-19 emergency?
    a. [If encouraged]: How frequently were patients encouraged to use V-safe?
    b. [If encouraged]: How did patients respond to this encouragement?
    c. [If encouraged]: What did patients like or dislike about V-safe?
5. [P] [If aware of VAERS] Did you or your patients ever make a report to VAERS during the COVID-19 emergency?
    a. [If yes]: What was that process like?
    b. Were there barriers or challenges for you to report to VAERS?
    c. From your perspective, what could be done to improve this reporting process?

Communication, Public Perception, and Influence

The next several questions focus on your experience with vaccine safety communications during the COVID-19 emergency.

6. [P] How and where did you and your colleagues get COVID-19 vaccine safety information during the COVID-19 emergency?
7. If you had questions regarding vaccine safety during the COVID-19 emergency, what resources did you use to get answers and did you know who to contact for answers?
8. [P] How confident are you or your colleagues in the trustworthiness of COVID-19 vaccine safety information provided by CDC?
    a. [If confident]: What factors have contributed to high confidence in COVID-19 vaccine safety information provided by CDC?

APPENDIX C

b. [If not confident]: What factors have contributed to low confidence in COVID-19 vaccine safety information provided by CDC?
c. [P] What could CDC do to increase confidence in COVID-19 vaccine safety information?
9. [P] From your perspective, how clear and timely were CDC's communications regarding COVID-19 vaccine safety during the COVID-19 emergency?
10. [P] From your perspective, how effectively does the CDC address public concerns about COVID-19 vaccine safety?
    a. How does your perception of CDC's effectiveness at addressing public concerns differ between during a public health emergency to other times?
11. What ways have patients shared they receive COVID-19 vaccine safety information?
    a. What ways have patients from marginalized groups shared they receive COVID-19 vaccine safety information?
    b. What improvements would you recommend for communicating COVID-19 vaccine safety information to patients, the public, and marginalized groups?

General Experience During Public Health Emergency and Suggestions for Improvement

Lastly, we'd like to learn about your overall experience with CDC's vaccine safety research and communications, and suggestions for improvement for the future.

12. [P] What is your overall perception of CDC's efforts pertaining to vaccine safety?
    a. What could the CDC do differently to enhance these efforts?
    b. What kinds of process improvements to vaccine safety systems, research, and communications would you recommend to the CDC?
13. [P] What do you think is the most important way to improve CDC's vaccine safety systems, research, and communications?
14. Is there anything else you'd like to share regarding your perspectives on vaccine safety as a healthcare professional?

Those are all the questions we have for you today. Thank you so much for taking the time to share your experiences and feedback. This concludes our discussion. Have a great rest of your day!

Outside Vaccine Safety Experts

Interviewee Role's

I'd like to start with brief introductions.

1. What is your area of expertise/profession?
2. What was your role or focus during the COVID-19 emergency (from March 2020 through May 2023)?

Perception of CDC ISO Vaccine Safety Research, Expertise, and Communications

Next, we'd like to learn about your perspectives regarding the CDC ISO's vaccine safety research focus areas, as well as the CDC ISO's capabilities and expertise. *[Research team – there may be limited understanding of CDC efforts vs. other agencies and we need to probe on responses to distinguish.]*

3. How do you view and balance different sources of vaccine safety research information?
4. How do you view the CDC ISO's vaccine safety research and communications?
    a. What are the strengths of or gaps in CDC ISO's vaccine safety research and communications?
    b. How has your perception of CDC ISO's vaccine safety research and communications changed since during the COVID-19 emergency to now?
5. How do you view the CDC ISO's vaccine safety capabilities and expertise?
    a. What are the strengths of or gaps in CDC ISO's vaccine safety capabilities and expertise?
    b. How has your perception of CDC ISO's vaccine safety capabilities and expertise changed since during the COVID-19 emergency to now?
6. From your perspective, does CDC ISO ask the right vaccine safety questions? Why or why not?
7. From your perspective, does CDC ISO have the necessary resources to research vaccine safety in a timely manner? Why or why not?

APPENDIX C

8. From your perspective, does the CDC ISO communicate their vaccine safety research results in a timely and appropriate manner? Why or why not?
9. What is your perspective on the issue of balancing informing the public about potential vaccine safety issues and providing the public with clear vaccine guidance?
    a. How well did the CDC ISO strike this balance during the COVID-19 emergency? How could the CDC ISO better address this balance?
10. How do you view CDC ISO's vaccine safety information in comparison to other sources?

Usage of CDC Data and Collaborations

Our next several questions focus on your experiences with the CDC ISO's vaccine safety data, as well as your collaborations and communications with the CDC ISO.

11. How have you used VAERS or VSD public data in your own vaccine safety research?
    a. How easy or difficult was it to use these data sources?
    b. What made these data sources easy or difficult to use?
    c. How could these data sources be improved?
12. How useful were the following resources to you during the COVID-19 emergency compared to now? [probe on each resource]
    a. V-safe
    b. CISA
    c. VAERS
    d. VSD
13. Outside the context of a public health emergency, how do you collaborate and communicate with CDC's ISO?
    a. How frequently do you try to use CDC ISO vaccine safety data?
    b. [If not mentioned]: How frequently do you collaborate with the CDC ISO?
    c. [If not mentioned]: What types of collaboration and communication do you have with CDC's ISO?
    d. What worked well in your collaboration with the CDC ISO?
    e. What could be improved in your collaboration with the CDC ISO?

General Experience During Public Health Emergency and Suggestions for Improvement

Lastly, we'd like to learn about your overall experience with CDC ISO's vaccine safety processes and communications, and suggestions for improvement for the future.

14. How can CDC ISO's vaccine safety systems, processes, research, and communications be improved going forward?
    a. How can the efficiency and effectiveness of vaccine safety data sharing be improved?
15. How can CDC ISO's vaccine safety processes and communications be improved to strengthen the public's confidence in vaccines?
    a. How can CDC's vaccine safety processes and communications be improved to strengthen marginalized groups' confidence in vaccines?
16. Is there anything else you'd like to share regarding your experiences regarding vaccine safety as a vaccine researcher during the COVID-19 emergency?

Those are all the questions we have for you today. Thank you so much for taking the time to share your experiences and feedback. This concludes our discussion. Have a great rest of your day!

Public Health Officials

Interviewee's Role

I'd like to start by learning about your role and experience. This is to help us interpret and analyze your responses. We will not directly cite or refer to your position in our summary report.

1. What is your position, and what are your current responsibilities?
2. What was your role during the COVID-19 emergency (from March 2020 through May 2023)?

Communication, Public Perception, and Influence

Next, we'd like to learn about your experiences as a [state, local, or tribal] public health official with vaccine safety communications during the COVID-19 emergency, starting in March 2020 through May 2023.

APPENDIX C *171*

3. [P] How and where did you get your COVID-19 vaccine safety messaging and talking points?
    a. [If not mentioned]: What resources from the CDC and other U.S. federal agencies did you use?
    b. [P] [If not mentioned]: Did you use the vaccine safety information contained on CDC's Interim Clinical recommendation for COVID-19 vaccines webpage or CDC HAN alerts?
        i. [If no]: Why did you not use these resources?
    c. Other than U.S. federal agencies, what sources did you use to find and communicate COVID-19 vaccine safety information?
        i. [If not mentioned]: Did you use messaging from vaccine manufacturers, other countries, or the World Health Organization? If so, which of these did you use?
        ii. [If yes]: If you used messaging from sources other than CDC and U.S. federal agencies, why did you use them?
    d. When your health department received questions about COVID-19 vaccine safety from healthcare providers or other groups, what resources did the health department use to answer these questions?
        i. [P] Did providers raise questions or concerns regarding information they were leveraging from CDC on vaccine safety?
4. [P] What feedback can you share about COVID-19 vaccine safety information or resources that you used from the CDC/<u>Advisory Committee on Immunization Practices</u> (ACIP)?
    a. What was your experience navigating these resources to find needed information and answer questions, especially considering when vaccine safety information recommendations evolved over time?
5. [P] What challenges did your health department encounter with regards to disinformation about COVID-19 vaccine safety?
    a. How useful were CDC's resources for addressing or clarifying issues?
6. [P] What types of additional vaccine safety communications support from CDC would have been helpful for your health department?
    a. [If not mentioned]: Which of the following resources would have been helpful: template presentations, handouts, job aids, FAQ documents, office hours, or others?

General Experience During Public Health Emergency and Suggestions for Improvement

Lastly, we'd like to learn about your overall experience with and perspective regarding vaccine safety information and communications.

7. What is your overall perception of CDC ISO's vaccine safety information?
8. [P] How, if at all, has your overall perception of CDC ISO's vaccine safety information changed from during the COVID-19 public health emergency to now?
9. [P] What factors do you consider when determining what vaccine safety information to share with the public?
   a. Which factors do you think are the most important in determining vaccine safety information to share with the public?
10. Is there anything else you'd like to share regarding your experiences with vaccine safety information during the COVID-19 emergency?

Those are all the questions we have for you today. Thank you so much for taking the time to share your experiences and feedback. This concludes our discussion. Have a great rest of your day.

APPENDIX B. RECRUITMENT LETTERS

Section A. Westat Recruitment Letters

Health Professionals, Vaccine Safety Experts, State and Local PH officials

To: X
Cc: Jennifer Edwards, Westat Project Director
Subject: [Response Requested]: Participation in NASEM/Westat interview on COVID-19 PHE experience

Dear X,

The Centers for Disease Control and Prevention (CDC) Immunization Safety Office (ISO) is sponsoring a study by the National Academies of Sciences, Engineering, and Medicine (NASEM) to evaluate COVID-19 vaccine safety research and communications during the public health emergency. Please see additional information about the study here:

APPENDIX C   173

Review of CDC COVID-19 Vaccine Safety Research and Communications | National Academies.

As a part of this study, NASEM and a NASEM appointed Committee would like to solicit input and feedback from government staff, researchers, healthcare professionals, and state and local health department officials about their experiences during the public health emergency (from December 2020 – May 2023) and perspectives on policies and procedures that worked or need improvement, collaboration and coordination, and communications about vaccine safety.

NASEM staff, in consult with the Committee, identified you as an expert in one or more of these topic areas. We are writing to see if you would be willing to participate in either a 60-minute one- on-one interview or a 90-minute focus group in January or February of 2025. To identify your interest or potential willingness to participate, we are providing a link below to a very brief survey (Please feel free to complete this from home as well if you prefer; please check your agency/organization IT policies before responding to ensure your privacy on those systems). In this survey, you can provide your preferred contact method, indicate your willingness to participate in either an interview of focus group, and answer a few questions to help us identify or confirm your areas of expertise. We may not be able to interview all interested participants.

This study is being carried out under the oversight of the NASEM IRB. Your participation in the study will be confidential – only Westat will have access to participant information and will not disclose the names, positions, or other identifying information of participants; all information to include your name, contact information, response to the survey, and subsequent interview material will be deleted. We will provide additional information regarding participant privacy and confidentiality during scheduling should you be selected to participate.

Link:
Password:
Participants can also access the survey via this QR code:

Please reach out to the Project Director, Jennifer Edwards, with any additional questions you may have.

Jennifer Edwards, PhD
Principal Investigator and Project Director, Westat

Sincerely, Neni Osuoha

Neni Osuoha, MPH, PMP (she, her, hers) Senior Research Associate I Westat Social Policy and Economic Research
1600 Research Blvd. I Rockville, MD 20850

CDC Staff, Funded Researchers, and other Govt Staff

To: X
Cc: Jennifer Edwards, Westat Project Director
Subject: Participation in NASEM/Westat interview on COVID-19 PHE experience Dear X,
The Centers for Disease Control and Prevents (CDC) Immunization Safety Office (ISO) is sponsoring a study by the National Academies of Sciences, Engineering, and Medicine (NASEM) to evaluate COVID-19 vaccine safety research and communications during the public health emergency. You should have received notification of this study in an email from Dr. Meyer on January 10th. See additional information about the study here: Review of CDC COVID-19 Vaccine Safety Research and Communications I National Academies.

As a part of this study, NASEM and a NASEM-appointed committee would like to solicit input and feedback from government staff, researchers, healthcare professionals, and state and local health department officials about their experiences during the public health emergency (from December 2020 – May 2023) and perspectives on policies and procedures that worked or need improvement, collaboration and coordination, and communications about vaccine safety.

NASEM staff, using publicly available information, identified you as an expert in one or more of these topic areas. We are writing to see if you would be willing to participate in a 60-minute one- on-one interview in January and February. To identify your interest or potential willingness to participate, we are providing a link below to a very brief survey. In this survey, you can provide your preferred contact method, indicate your willingness to participate, and answer a few questions to help us identify or confirm your areas of expertise. We may not be able to interview all willing participants.

APPENDIX C   175

This study is being carried out with the oversight of the NASEM IRB. Your participation in the study will not be disclosed to CDC staff, NASEM staff, or the Committee and all information to include your name, contact information, response to the survey, and subsequent interview material will be deleted. To further ensure your privacy, please refer to agency IT policies before using your official email to respond or choosing your method of response as communications on federal systems may be subject to FOIA requests. We provide additional information regarding participant privacy and confidentiality on the survey site.

Link:
Password:
Participants can also access the survey via this QR code:

Please reach out to the Project Director, Jennifer Edwards, with any additional questions you may have.
Jennifer Edwards, PhD
Principal Investigator and Project Director, Westat

Sincerely, Neni Osuoha

Neni Osuoha, MPH, PMP (she, her, hers) Senior Research Associate I Westat Social Policy and Economic Research
1600 Research Blvd. I Rockville, MD 20850

APPENDIX C. INFORMED CONSENT

Individual Interview Informed Consent Form

Purpose of Study

In early 2024, the Centers for Disease Control and Prevention (CDC) Immunization Safety Office (ISO) asked the National Academies of Sciences, Engineering, and Medicine (NASEM) to conduct a consensus study to evaluate the systems, methods, and processes for monitoring COVID-19 vaccine safety during the U.S. COVID-19 public health emergency, and provide recommendations for sustaining, maintaining, and strengthening CDC ISO current monitoring systems and communications moving forward.

Westat was contracted by NASEM's Health and Medicine Division (HMD) to conduct this study for the CDC. Our purpose is to conduct confidential interviews with key informants regarding the ISO's research on

COVID-19 vaccine safety and communications about COVID-19 vaccine safety during the public health emergency (PHE). The findings from these interviews will be analyzed and summarized for inclusion in a publicly available report produced by NASEM.

Participant Selection

You were identified by NASEM staff and NASEM appointed committee members as knowledgeable about the CDC ISO's systems, methods, and processes for monitoring COVID-19 vaccine safety. You completed a participant screening form and were selected to participate in a 60-minute interview for this study. Although NASEM identified potential study participants, Westat will not disclose participants names to NASEM or CDC.

Study Procedure

Depending on your role, we may ask you questions about three general topic areas regarding CDC vaccine safety research and communications during the COVID-19 emergency: (1) policies and procedures; (2) interagency collaboration and coordination; and (3) communication and public perception.

To confirm your knowledge of these topics, the brief recruitment survey asks you to confirm your professional affiliation (where you work) now at and at the time of the COVID-19 public health emergency as well as your familiarity with or use of ISO information. It also asks for your preferred contact method. If selected for an interview, we will reach out to schedule that interview. Once completed, survey responses including your contact information and name are destroyed. If not selected, your survey response and contact information will also be removed/destroyed.

Following completion of your interview, conducted via Zoom and recorded (if you agree), we will transcribe the interview and redact any potentially identifiable information. At that time, the recording of your interview will also be destroyed as will the unredacted transcript. The redacted transcript will be retained on Westat secure systems until the report is published and then will be destroyed.

Benefits

There will be no direct benefit to you for your participation in the study. An indirect benefit of your participation will be the knowledge that your input was invaluable and contributed to strengthening future CDC vaccine monitoring systems and communication efforts.

Risks and Discomfort & Privacy and Confidentiality

The potential risks to participation in this study may vary based on the role and affiliation of the participant, with government employees facing additional professional risks potentially due to the high level of public interest in the topic and the potential for FOIA requests in regard to the study. While our procedures minimize this risk and there is an exemption category to a FOIA request that should apply here (category 6), we cannot completely eliminate risk. We recognize conversations about vaccine safety and the COVID-19 emergency can be politically sensitive and reflecting on that time period can cause emotional discomfort. The information you provide will only be used for the research purposes of this study and it will be handled in a private and confidential manner. What we discuss will not be shared with your colleagues at any level or the public. Please be advised that we may include paraphrases of comments made in the report, but these will not be attributed to your name or position title.

We would like to record the interview for notetaking purposes only with your permission. You may decide not to be recorded, pause the recording, or stop the recording altogether at any time. All study materials, including the meeting recording, transcript, and notes will be stored on Westat's secure server and will only be accessible to the Westat staff working on this study. Any sensitive material, including personally identifiable information (PII), will be redacted from interview transcripts and notes. Participant names and contact information, including Qualtrics survey responses, will be destroyed upon interview completion. Interview recordings will be deleted upon review and redaction of PII from transcripts and notes. All other data, such as transcripts and analytic files, will be destroyed after the overall study is completed and published.

Study Costs and Compensation

There are no costs for your participation in this study apart from the time you spend with us for this interview. There is no monetary compensation for your participation in this study.

Voluntary Participation

Your participation in the interview as well as responding to individual interview questions is voluntary. You may decide not to participate, and it will not have any impact on your position. You may take a break, skip questions, speak off the record, or stop participating at any time.

More Information

If you have any questions or would like more information about this study, please contact Jennifer Edwards, the study Project Director, at 1-301-212-3216. If you have questions about your rights and welfare as a research participant, please call the NASEM Institutional Review Board office at 202.334.1616. Please leave a message with your full name, the name of the research study that you are calling about (Key Informant Interviews for the National Academies' Health and Medicine Division), and a phone number beginning with the area code. Someone will return your call as soon as possible.

Certification of Informed Consent

We will ask you to verbally consent to participate in the study and confirm you have reviewed this agreement during the interview.

Focus Group Informed Consent Form

Purpose of Study

In early 2024, the Centers for Disease Control and Prevention (CDC) Immunization Safety Office (ISO) asked the National Academies of Sciences, Engineering, and Medicine (NASEM) to conduct a consensus study to evaluate the systems, methods, and processes for monitoring COVID-19 vaccine safety during the U.S. COVID-19 public health emergency, and provide recommendations for sustaining, maintaining, and strengthening CDC ISO current monitoring systems and communications moving forward.

Westat was contracted by NASEM's Health and Medicine Division (HMD) to conduct this study for the CDC. Our purpose is to conduct confidential interviews with key informants regarding the ISO's research on COVID-19 vaccine safety and communications about COVID-19 vaccine safety during the public health emergency (PHE). The findings from these interviews will be analyzed and summarized for inclusion in a report produced by NASEM.

Participant Selection

You were identified by NASEM staff and NASEM appointed committee members as knowledgeable about the CDC ISO's systems, methods, and processes for monitoring COVID-19 vaccine safety. You completed a participant screening form and were selected to participate in a 90-minute focus group for this study. Although NASEM identified potential study

APPENDIX C   *179*

participants, Westat will not disclose participants' names to NASEM or CDC or any other entity.

Study Procedure

Depending on your role, we may ask you questions about three general topic areas regarding CDC vaccine safety research and communications during the COVID-19 emergency: (1) policies and procedures; (2) inter-agency collaboration and coordination; and (3) communication and public perception.

To confirm your knowledge of these topics, the brief recruitment survey asks you to confirm your professional affiliation (where you work) now at and at the time of the COVID-19 public health emergency as well as your familiarity with or use of ISO information. It also asks for your preferred contact method. If selected for a focus group, we will reach out to schedule that. Once completed, survey responses including your contact information and name are destroyed. If not selected, your survey response and contact information will also be removed/destroyed.

Following completion of your focus group, conducted via Zoom and recorded (if all agree), we will transcribe the session and redact any potentially identifiable information. At that time, the recording of your session will also be destroyed as will the unredacted transcript. The redacted transcript will be retained on Westat secure systems until the report is published and then will be destroyed.

Benefits

There will be no direct benefit to you for your participation in the study. An indirect benefit of your participation will be the knowledge that your input was invaluable and contributed to strengthening future CDC vaccine monitoring systems and communication efforts.

Risks and Discomfort & Privacy and Confidentiality

The potential risks to participation in this study may vary based on the role and affiliation of the participant. We recognize conversations about vaccine safety and the COVID-19 emergency can be politically sensitive and reflecting on that time period can cause emotional discomfort. We encourage you to only answer questions you feel comfortable responding to. There is no obligation to respond to each question. To facilitate information sharing, the focus group will also use a tool/platform that enables anonymous responses. The information you provide will only be used for the research purposes of this study and it will be handled in a private and confidential manner. Please be advised that we may include paraphrases of your statements in the report, but these will not be attributed to your name or position title.

Because this is a focus group the other participants will of course be aware of your feedback and you will be aware of theirs. We will remind all participants to respect the privacy of each other and not disclose individuals' feedback. However, disclosure from other participants is a risk.

We would like to record the session with your permission. All study materials, including the meeting recording, transcript, and notes will be stored on Westat's secure server and will only be accessible to the Westat staff working on this study. Any sensitive material, including personally identifiable information (PII), will be redacted from interview transcripts and notes. Participant names and contact information, including Qualtrics survey responses, will be destroyed upon interview completion. Interview recordings will be deleted upon review and redaction of PII from transcripts and notes. All other data, such as transcripts and analytic files, will be destroyed after the overall study is completed and published.

Study Costs and Compensation

There are no costs for your participation in this study apart from the time you spend with us for this interview. There is no monetary compensation for your participation in this study.

Voluntary Participation

Your participation in the interview as well as responding to individual interview questions is voluntary. You may decide not to participate, and it will not have any impact on your position. You may take a break, skip questions, speak off the record, or stop participating at any time.

More Information

If you have any questions or would like more information about this study, please contact Jennifer Edwards, the study Project Director. If you have questions about your rights and welfare as a research participant, please call the NASEM Institutional Review Board office at 202.334.1616. Please leave a message with your full name, the name of the research study that you are calling about (Key Informant Interviews for the National Academies' Health and Medicine Division), and a phone number beginning with the area code. Someone will return your call as soon as possible.

Certification of Informed Consent

We will ask you to verbally consent to participate in the study and confirm you have reviewed this document at the start of the focus group.

Appendix D

Case Studies

INTRODUCTION

The goal of these case studies is to illustrate how the Centers for Disease Control and Prevention (CDC) identified, assessed, and communicated adverse events (AEs) associated with COVID vaccines. They highlight both prespecified AEs and those that emerged during the vaccination campaign, offering insight into the Immunization Safety Office (ISO) approach to vaccine safety monitoring and response. The case studies focus on three specific AEs linked to vaccination: myocarditis, tinnitus, and menstrual irregularities. Myocarditis was identified early as an adverse event of special interest (AESI); the latter two emerged as concerns through postmarketing surveillance and public reports. Additionally, a brief case study on the chikungunya vaccine is included as a real-time example of how vaccine safety monitoring continues to evolve beyond the COVID response.

The case studies were developed using publicly available information from the COVID-19 Vaccine Safety Technical (VaST) Work Group and Advisory Committee on Immunization Practices (ACIP), primarily sourced through the CDC Stacks archive website during the time of the U.S. public health emergency (PHE). Publications and public presentations to this committee from ISO were also used. While these sources provide valuable insights into ISO's and CDC's safety monitoring and communication strategies, there are inherent limitations. These case studies rely exclusively on publicly available data, which means they may not fully capture all internal deliberations, emerging evidence, or evolving risk assessments conducted within CDC and its partner agencies. Despite this limitation, these case studies offer a useful perspective on ISO's vaccine safety efforts and highlight key lessons for future vaccine monitoring, regulatory decision making, and public health communication strategies.

MYOCARDITIS CASE STUDY

Myocarditis is an inflammatory condition that affects the myocardium or heart muscle (Ammirati et al., 2020). It can result from an infection, immune system response, or drug exposure, prompting immune activation, inflammation in the heart muscle, and heart cell damage (Ammirati et al., 2020; Nagai et al., 2023). Acute myocarditis frequently presents with nonspecific signs and symptoms, such as chest pain, dyspnea, or palpitations. It most often affects people aged 30–45, with men making up 60–80 percent of cases (Ammirati and Moslehi, 2023; Basso, 2022). Globally, myocarditis occurs in about 4–14 people per 100,000 each year, though the actual rate is likely higher due to many mild or undiagnosed cases (Ammirati and Moslehi, 2023; Nagai et al., 2023). Outcomes vary depending on the disease cause and form, with reported death rates for acute myocarditis of 1–7 percent (Ammirati and Moslehi, 2023; Nagai et al., 2023).

Myocarditis was not reported as a postvaccination event in the clinical trial data for BNT162b2 (Pfizer-BioNTech), mRNA-1273 (Moderna), or Ad26.COV2.S (Janssen) vaccines that were granted initial emergency use authorization, according to Baden et al. (2021), Polack et al. (2020), and Sadoff et al. (2021). However, myocarditis was designated as an AESI for the COVID vaccine in the United States (VAERS, n.d.) due to its association with the COVID disease pathology and potential to signal vaccine-associated enhanced disease (VAED).

The case definition of myocarditis developed by the ACIP Joint Smallpox Vaccine Safety Working Group and Armed Forced Epidemiology Board (AFEB) during the 2002–2003 vaccination campaign for military personnel and civilian health care and public health professionals in response to a bioterrorism threat (CDC, 2003; Poland et al., 2005) was adopted for monitoring during the COVID vaccination effort (CDC, 2003; VAERS, n.d.). Myopericarditis was an unexpected AE from the live smallpox vaccine used in the campaign (Poland et al., 2005). An incidence of 16.11 per 100,000 vaccine recipients was observed among military personnel (Arness et al., 2004; Poland et al., 2005). It was concluded that the smallpox vaccination appeared to increase the risk in recipients, particularly among men (Poland et al., 2005). Aside from these cases, myocarditis is rarely reported to the Vaccine Adverse Event Reporting System (VAERS) or in the literature as a vaccine-related AE (Mei et al., 2018; Montgomery et al., 2021).

Event Timeline

As it was an AESI, multiple vaccine safety systems were used to proactively monitor for myocarditis once U.S. COVID vaccinations commenced, including several ISO systems, specifically VAERS and the Vaccine Safety Datalink (VSD) (Gee et al., 2024; Markowitz et al., 2024). VaST routinely reviewed data on AESIs, including myocarditis, to make a benefit–risk assessment. The Vaccine Safety Team (VST) reported safety monitoring data, and VaST reported its risk assessments to the ACIP COVID-19 Vaccines Work Group and ACIP. VST reported that no safety signals had been detected related to myocarditis at the ACIP meetings on January 27, 2021 and March 1, 2021 based on interim analyses of VSD rapid-cycle analysis (RCA) (Shimabukuro, 2021c). The VSD RCA used data on AESIs reported weekly by nine participating integrated health care organizations to monitor for potential safety signals. Table D-1 presents a timeline summarizing the events related to the initial safety signal detection through ACIP determination and communication.

Initial Signal Detection

The first signs of a potential safety concern related to myocarditis emerged in spring 2021 (Gee et al., 2024). In February 2021, the Ministry of Health in Israel began active monitoring for myocarditis after receipt of the Pfizer-BioNTech vaccine based on reports from HCPs (Mevorach et al., 2021). All hospitals were asked to report myocarditis cases; 142 were reported following COVID vaccination from December 2020 through May 2021. The incidence was greatest among boys and men after the second dose.

In the United States, the first signal was detected within the military population based on referrals to the Defense Health Agency clinical specialists and VAERS reports (Gee et al., 2024; Montgomery et al., 2021). Between January and April 2021, the military administered 2.8 million vaccine doses, and 23 men were evaluated and diagnosed with myocarditis following mRNA COVID vaccination (Montgomery et al., 2021). Twenty of these cases occurred following the second vaccine dose. The Pfizer-BioNTech vaccine was authorized for individuals aged ≥ 16 and adolescents aged 12–15, while the Moderna and Janssen vaccines were authorized for persons aged ≥ 18 (CDC, 2024).

TABLE D-1 Timeline of Events Related to Signal Detection of Myocarditis Following U.S. mRNA COVID Vaccination

Date	Vaccine Authorization/ Approval and Recommendation	Myocarditis Signal Detection
December 11, 2020	FDA issues EUA for Pfizer-BioNTech vaccine; ACIP recommends for people aged ≥16 (CDC, 2024)	
December 14, 2020	First COVID vaccine administered (Guarino et al., 2020)	
December 18–19, 2020	FDA issues EUA for Moderna vaccine; ACIP recommends for people aged ≥18 (CDC, 2024)	
January 27, 2021		VST reports no safety signal detected for myocarditis in VAERS or VSD at ACIP meeting (Shimabukuro, 2021c)
February 27–28, 2021	FDA issues EUA for Janssen vaccine; ACIP recommends for people aged ≥18 (CDC, 2024)	
February 2021		Israeli Ministry of Health begins active monitoring for myocarditis after the Pfizer-BioNTech vaccine (Mevorach et al., 2021)
March 1, 2021		VST reports no safety signal detected for myocarditis in VAERS or VSD at ACIP meeting (Shimabukuro, 2021c)
April 2021		VaST first discusses myocarditis as a safety concern following mRNA vaccination (Markowitz et al., 2024)
May 10–12, 2021	FDA expands Pfizer-BioNTech vaccine EUA; ACIP recommends for adolescents aged 12–15 (CDC, 2024)	
May 17, 2021		VaST issues report on myocarditis following mRNA vaccination[a,b] (NCIRD, 2021a)

TABLE D-1 Continued

Date	Vaccine Authorization/ Approval and Recommendation	Myocarditis Signal Detection
May 24, 2021		VaST issues report on myocarditis following mRNA vaccination[c,d] (NCIRD, 2021c)
May 2021		VaST issues clinical guidance to HCPs on the assessment and treatment of myocarditis (ACIP, 2021a; Shimabukuro, 2021d)
June 23, 2021		ACIP issues determination on myocarditis following mRNA vaccination and initiates a study to evaluate the long-term outcomes[e] (Gargano, 2021)
June 25, 2021		FDA revises the EUAs and fact sheets for the Pfizer-BioNTech and Moderna vaccines with information about myocarditis (ACIP, 2021a)
July 9, 2021		MMWR publishes ACIP determination on myocarditis risk from June 23, 2021 meeting (Gargano, 2021)
August 13, 2021	ACIP recommends an additional dose of vaccine after the two-dose primary series for moderately to severely compromised individuals (CDC, 2024)	
August 23–30, 2021	FDA fully approves the Pfizer-BioNTech vaccine for people 18+; ACIP recommends for people 16+ (CDC, 2024)	
August 2021		CDC launches follow-up study on long-term outcomes of myocarditis after mRNA vaccine (Kracalik et al., 2022)

[a] Concluded that the rate of myocarditis reports following mRNA COVID vaccination was consistent with expected baseline rates; however, cases seemed to occur more frequently in adolescents and young adults, boys and men, following the second dose, and within 4 days following vaccination.

continued

TABLE D-1 Continued

^{b} Recommended ongoing monitoring of reported myocarditis cases, education for HCPs to support timely identification and proper management, and the development of clinical guidance on diagnosis and treatment.
  ^{c} Continued to support ongoing monitoring of reported cases, particularly in younger age groups, HCP education, and the development of clinical guidance.
  ^{d} Advocated for follow-up of individuals with myocarditis following COVID vaccination to understand long-term outcomes.
  ^{e} Determination: "… the benefits of using mRNA COVID-19 vaccines under the FDA's EUA clearly outweigh the risks in all populations, including adolescents and young adults."
NOTE: ACIP = Advisory Committee on Immunization Practices; EUA = emergency use authorization; FDA = Food and Drug Administration; HCP = health care provider; VAERS = Vaccine Adverse Event Reporting System; VaST = Vaccine Safety Technical (a work group); VSD = Vaccine Safety Datalink; VST = Vaccine Safety Team.

VaST Review

VaST first discussed the myocarditis as a safety concern after mRNA COVID vaccination in April 2021 (Markowitz et al., 2024). On May 17, 2021, its meeting included updates on myocarditis reports following mRNA vaccination from VAERS and VSD, among other vaccine safety monitoring systems (NCIRD, 2021a). VaST concluded that the rate of reports was consistent with expected baseline rates. Among the limited number of cases, myocarditis seemed to occur more frequently in adolescents and young adults, boys and men, following the second dose, and within 4 days of vaccination. VaST recommended ongoing monitoring of reported cases, education for HCPs to support timely identification and proper management, and the development of clinical guidance on diagnosis and treatment.

On May 24, 2021, the VaST meeting included updates on myocarditis following mRNA vaccination (NCIRD, 2021c). VAERS data indicated that reports were higher than expected among 16–24-year-old individuals within 30 days of the second dose. VSD data showed no difference in the rates of myocarditis following mRNA vaccination compared to expected rates. VaST continued to support ongoing monitoring of reported cases, particularly in younger age groups, HCP education, and the development of clinical guidance and advocated for ongoing monitoring of individuals who were affected to understand long-term outcomes.

ACIP Determination

The ACIP meeting on June 23, 2021 focused on myocarditis after mRNA vaccination (ACIP, 2021b). Speakers presented an overview of myocarditis, updates from the COVID-19 VST, and VaST's assessment (Lee and

Hopkins, 2021; Oster, 2021b; Shimabukuro, 2021d; Wallace and Oliver, 2021). As of June 11, 2021, VAERS had received 791 reports following administration of the Pfizer-BioNTech vaccine (150 after the first dose and 563 after the second) and 435 reports following the Moderna vaccine (117 after the first dose and 264 after the second), when approximately 300 million mRNA vaccine doses had been administered (ACIP, 2021b; Shimabukuro, 2021d). The highest number of reports occurred after the second dose, predominantly among individuals in their late teens to mid-20s, and typically within 7 days of vaccination.

As of June 12, 2021, the VSD rapid cycle analysis (RCA) detected no statistical signal for myocarditis or pericarditis within 21 days after either dose of an mRNA vaccine, with an adjusted rate ratio slightly above 1 (ACIP, 2021b; Shimabukuro, 2021d). An age-stratified analysis of individuals aged 12–39 identified a statistically significant increase in myocarditis cases within 21 days of receiving an mRNA vaccine, with a combined adjusted rate ratio of 3.5. The increased risk was significant after the second dose but not the first. Estimates for the Pfizer-BioNTech vaccine did not reach significance. Thus, the overall findings were likely influenced by cases associated with the Moderna vaccine, despite limited data for control comparisons. A similar analysis using a 7-day risk window yielded comparable findings. VaST concluded that current evidence supported a likely link between mRNA COVID vaccination and myocarditis in adolescents and young adults, particularly among boys and men and after the second dose (ACIP, 2021b; Lee and Hopkins, 2021). These cases typically presented within 1 week postvaccination and were consistent across both VAERS and VSD data, strengthening confidence in the observed patterns.

The ACIP COVID-19 Work Group presented a benefit–risk framework that included consideration of the following benefits: COVID-19 cases prevented, COVID-19 hospitalizations prevented, and COVID-19 intensive care unit (ICU) admissions and deaths prevented (Gargano, 2021). Risks included the number of myocarditis reports to VAERs within 7 days after a second dose of an mRNA vaccine. The benefits and risks were assessed across various age cohorts and sex. At the population level, the absence of alternative vaccines for adolescents was considered. ACIP concluded that the benefits of mRNA vaccination still outweighed the risks for adolescents and young adults based on available data related to myocarditis (ACIP, 2021b; Gargano, 2021). The ACIP conclusion also affirmed the importance of continuing to monitor myocarditis outcomes and providing education to HCPs and the public. To monitor, CDC initiated a study with follow-up on myocarditis reports to VAERS (Kracalik, 2022).

Public and Provider Communication

CDC used multiple strategies to communicate information regarding myocarditis after mRNA COVID vaccination to the public and HCPs. In May 2021, VaST issued clinical guidance to HCPs on assessing and treating myocarditis via the "Clinical Considerations: Myocarditis and Pericarditis after Receipt of mRNA COVID-19 Vaccines Among Adolescents and Young Adults" webpage (CDC, 2023b) and a webpage with clinical guidance regarding administration of a second dose in people who developed myocarditis after the first dose (ACIP, 2021a; Gargano, 2021; Shimabukuro, 2021d).

Furthermore, a summary of ACIP's determination from the June 23rd meeting and rationale were published in MMWR on July 9, 2021 (Gargano, 2021). Beyond CDC's communication efforts, the Food and Drug Administration (FDA) revised the Pfizer-BioNTech and Moderna COVID vaccine EUAs and fact sheets with information about myocarditis on June 25, 2021 (Gargano, 2021; Lee and Hopkins, 2021; Markowitz et al., 2024).

The webpage "Myocarditis and Pericarditis Following mRNA COVID-19 Vaccination," summarized key information for the public, including CDC's ongoing recommendation that all individuals 12+ years be vaccinated and what symptoms to monitor for afterward (NCIRD, 2021f). Information about the risk of myocarditis after mRNA vaccination was added to CDC's webpages about the Pfizer-BioNTech and Moderna vaccines (Gargano, 2021; NCIRD, 2021e,h). Several additional webpages were updated to educate the public about myocarditis after mRNA vaccination, including "Selected adverse events reported after COVID-19 vaccination," "COVID-19 Vaccines That Require 2 Shots," and "COVID-19 Vaccines for Children and Teens" (NCIRD, 2021b,i).

Ongoing Monitoring

While ACIP's determination that the benefits of mRNA COVID vaccination outweighed the risk of myocarditis remained unchanged and vaccination continued to be recommended, cases of myocarditis after mRNA vaccination were continuously monitored through vaccine safety systems and regularly presented at ACIP meetings throughout the PHE (see Table D-2).

Myocarditis Long-Term Outcomes Study

In August 2021, CDC launched a follow-up study to examine clinical recovery and quality-of-life outcomes following an mRNA COVID vaccine (Kracalik et al., 2022). The study focused on patients aged 12–29 years

TABLE D-2 ACIP Meetings Addressing Myocarditis Following mRNA COVID Vaccination During the Public Health Emergency

Meeting Date	Summary
June 23, 2021	This was the first ACIP meeting focused on myocarditis after mRNA COVID vaccination (ACIP, 2021b). As of June 11, 2021, VAERS had received 791 reports following administration of the Pfizer-BioNTech vaccine and 435 reports following the Moderna vaccine out of approximately 300 million mRNA doses administered. As of June 12, 2021, a VSD age-stratified analysis of individuals aged 12–39 identified a statistically significant increase in cases within 21 days of receiving an mRNA vaccine, with a combined adjusted rate ratio of 3.5, likely influenced by cases associated with the Moderna vaccine. ACIP concluded that the benefits of mRNA vaccination still outweighed the risks for adolescents and young adults based on available data related to myocarditis. To monitor outcomes, CDC initiated a study with follow-up on myocarditis reports to VAERS.
August 30, 2021	Updated VAERS and VSD data were presented after FDA's approval of the Pfizer-BioNTech vaccine for individuals 18+ (ACIP, 2021a). As of August 18, VAERS had 1,903 reports of myocarditis, with patterns remaining consistent with previously reported data—most in younger male recipients shortly after the second dose of an mRNA vaccine. No safety signals were detected in the overall VSD population (≥12 years), but in individuals aged 12–39, both mRNA vaccines were linked to higher rates of myocarditis, particularly within the first week following vaccination. VaST presented its evaluation, indicating that the data suggest a link between myocarditis and mRNA vaccination in adolescents and young adults. ACIP voted to recommend the Pfizer-BioNTech vaccine, now fully approved, for individuals aged 16+, as a 30-microgram dose.

continued

TABLE D-2 Continued

Meeting Date	Summary
September 22–23, 2021	VaST presented on a potential third dose of the Pfizer-BioNTech vaccine (ACIP, 2021c). Data from Israel as of September 13, 2021, reported only a single case of myocarditis—a man in his 30s—after approximately 2.8 million third doses for individuals aged 12+. As a result of limitations in the available data, VaST outlined a plan to continue monitoring and reviewing safety data related to third doses. ACIP voted to recommend a 30-microgram third dose of the Pfizer-BioNTech vaccine for individuals 65+, residents of long-term care facilities, those aged 50–64 with underlying medical conditions, and individuals aged 18–49 with underlying medical conditions based on an individual benefit–risk assessment, all to be administered at least 6 months after completion of the primary series.
October 21, 2021	VST presented updated data on myocarditis (Shimabukuro and ACIP, 2021). VAERS data showed that 402,469,096 doses had been administered as of October 6, 2021, resulting in 2,459 reports of myopericarditis (Su, 2021b). The patterns of myocarditis after vaccination were consistent with prior reports. VSD indicated that both mRNA vaccines were linked to an increased risk in individuals aged 18–39, with the Pfizer-BioNTech vaccine also showing a higher risk in those aged 12–17 (Klein, 2021). Head-to-head comparisons suggested that the risk of myocarditis was greater after the Moderna compared to the Pfizer-BioNTech vaccine. The VaST assessment noted that safety data for the reduced 50-microgram Moderna booster dose were based on a small clinical trial and that the risk after this booster might be lower than that associated with the original, 100-microgram dose (Talbot and Hopkins, 2021). ACIP voted to recommend Pfizer-BioNTech and Moderna third doses to individuals 65+ years and those 18+ years who live in long-term care settings, have underlying medical conditions, or work or live in high-risk settings, all at least 6 months after completion of the primary series (CDC, 2021b).

TABLE D-2 Continued

Meeting Date	Summary
November 2, 2021	Updated VAERS and VSD data regarding myocarditis in individuals aged 12+ were presented (Oster, 2021a). The plans to use safety monitoring systems to track myocarditis, along with VaST's plan to review data for individuals aged 5–11 years, were also shared (Shimabukuro, 2021b). Key counseling points for HCPs regarding the risk in children aged 5–11 were highlighted: the benefits of vaccination outweigh the risks; individuals should seek medical care if they experience chest pain, shortness of breath, or elevated heart rate after an mRNA vaccine; no cases of myocarditis were reported in clinical trials for this age group; the risk is higher in adolescents aged 12–17 than in younger children; and the risk after mRNA vaccination is lower than that associated with COVID infection in adolescents and adults (Woodworth, 2021). It was discussed that the rate of myocarditis after vaccination in this age group was not yet known, but it was expected to be lower than in 12–15-year-olds due to the lower dose and observed epidemiologic differences in viral myocarditis between the two age groups (Oliver, 2021). ACIP recommended the Pfizer-BioNTech vaccine for all children ages 5–11, as a two-dose series of 10 micrograms each (CDC, 2024).
November 19, 2021	The VST presented updated VAERS data on reports following booster doses (Shimabukuro, 2021a). There were 54 preliminary reports of myocarditis and myopericarditis, aligning with the recommended booster dose population (e.g., adults over 65). VaST assessment noted that the risk appeared lower after a booster dose of the Pfizer-BioNTech vaccine compared to dose two of the primary series based on data from Israel (Talbot and Hopkins, 2022c). There was insufficient data to assess the myocarditis risk following a Moderna booster dose. Accumulating evidence indicating a higher myocarditis risk after the Moderna primary series compared to Pfizer-BioNTech was noted; however, the Moderna booster was a lower dose than the primary series (50 micrograms vs. 100 micrograms). ACIP expanded the recommendation for a booster dose to all individuals $\geq$18 years (CDC, 2021a).
December 16, 2021	ACIP heard updates on AEs being reported to VAERS and VSD in children aged 5–11 following the COVID vaccination primary series (Su, 2021a). Fourteen cases of myocarditis were reported to VAERS, eight of which had been verified, with no confirmed cases in VSD in the 7 and 21 days following vaccination.

continued

TABLE D-2 Continued

Meeting Date	Summary
January 5, 2022	VST presented updated VAERS and VSD data on myocarditis (ACIP, 2022b). As of December 19, 2021, VAERS had 265 confirmed myocarditis reports following Pfizer-BioNTech vaccine administration among children and adolescents ages 12–15 out of 18.7 million doses. There were 12 confirmed reports among children ages 5–11 out of 8.7 million doses and 13 preliminary reports of myocarditis following booster vaccination among adults 16–24 with approximately 1 million doses. VSD data continued to demonstrate an elevated risk of myocarditis in 12–17-year-olds in the 7 days following dose 2. The excess risk was 70 cases per million second doses compared to 0.3 cases per million first doses. Data from Israel on myocarditis reports after a third dose in children aged 12–15 years were also presented. No cases were reported with over 6,000 vaccine doses administered. ACIP voted to recommend a 30-microgram booster dose of the Pfizer-BioNTech vaccine in adolescents 12–17 years at least 5 months after completion of the primary series.
February 4, 2022	Updated VAERS data on myocarditis following administration of the Moderna vaccine, along with findings from the VSD RCA and a head-to-head comparison of mRNA vaccines, were presented. As of January 13, 2022, 359 myocarditis cases that met the case definition had been reported to VAERS among individuals 18+ within 7 days after Moderna vaccination, out of 164 million doses (Shimabukuro, 2022b). The VSD analysis with vaccinated concurrent comparators continued to show both mRNA vaccines were associated with increased risk of myocarditis in 18–39-year-olds (Klein, 2022). A head-to-head comparison of the vaccines using VSD data provided evidence that the risk of myocarditis may be higher after the Moderna vaccine compared to the Pfizer-BioNTech. VaST reported that its evaluation of updated data did not indicate any safety concerns related to myocarditis following the Moderna vaccine in individuals 18+ years beyond those already recognized (Talbot and Hopkins, 2022a).

TABLE D-2 Continued

Meeting Date	Summary
April 20, 2022	Updated data from VSD and VAERS on the safety of the first booster doses were presented (ACIP, 2022a). As of April 11, 2022, there were 100 cases of myocarditis in VAERS following a first mRNA COVID vaccine booster dose out of 93 million doses. Reporting rates were highest among male recipients ages 12–29, exceeding background rates but lower than those observed after the second dose of the primary series. The only safety signal noted after a first booster dose in VSD was myocarditis, primarily occurring within a week after a first booster dose in individuals aged 12–39. The VaST assessment was that the risk following a booster dose continued to appear lower than after the second dose of the primary series.
May 19, 2022	VST updated ACIP on myocarditis reports following the Pfizer-BioNTech primary series in children aged 5–11 (Shimabukuro, 2022a). As of April 24, 2022, 20 verified cases were reported in VAERS, out of 18.1 million doses, primarily after the second dose. The VSD RCA did not detect a statistically significant safety signal. VaST concluded that the data did not indicate any safety concerns with the Pfizer-BioNTech booster dose for children aged 5–11 beyond those already identified in older age groups (Talbot and Hopkins, 2022b). ACIP voted in favor of recommending the booster dose for this age group (ACIP, 2022e).
June 17–18, 2022	Representatives from Moderna and Pfizer presented updates on the effectiveness and safety of both mRNA COVID vaccines from clinical trials for young children (ACIP, 2022d). Myocarditis was not reported during clinical trials for either vaccine. The ACIP COVID-19 Work Group concluded that both the Moderna and Pfizer-BioNTech mRNA COVID vaccines for young children had favorable safety profiles, with common mild to moderate side effects similar to other routine childhood vaccines. ACIP voted to recommend the Moderna vaccine as a two-dose primary series of 25 micrograms per dose for children aged 6 months to 5 years and the Pfizer-BioNTech vaccine as a three-dose primary series of 3 micrograms per dose for children aged 6 months to 4 years.

continued

TABLE D-2 Continued

Meeting Date	Summary
June 23, 2022	VST presented updated data from VAERS and VSD on myocarditis in children and adolescents aged 6–11 and 12–17 following primary series vaccination with Pfizer-BioNTech (ACIP, 2022g). As of May 26, 2022, VAERS had 635 verified myocarditis reports among 5–17-year-olds out of 54.8 million doses. No safety signals were present in VSD for myocarditis in children aged 5–11; however, people ≥12 years had a statistically significant safety signal for both the primary series and booster doses. A head-to-head comparison of the two mRNA COVID vaccines in individuals aged 18–39 using VSD data provided evidence that the risk of myocarditis may be higher following the Moderna vaccine. The VaST assessment noted a risk of myocarditis after mRNA COVID vaccination in adolescents and adults, with ongoing evaluation and monitoring in children under 12. ACIP voted favorably to recommend the Moderna vaccine as a two-dose series of 50 micrograms per dose in children aged 6–11 and a two-dose series of 100 micrograms per dose in children and adolescents aged 12–17.
July 19, 2022	VST gave an update on myocarditis following mRNA COVID vaccination in adults ≥18 years based on VAERS and VSD data (ACIP, 2022c). As of May 26, 2022, VAERS had 1,321 verified myocarditis reports in individuals 18+ after 491.9 million doses. Evidence continued to show consistent patterns with previously reported data: cases were most likely within the first week postvaccination, with the highest risk in male adolescents and young adults, particularly after the second dose of the primary series.
September 1, 2022	VST presented on the safety of the primary series with a mRNA COVID vaccine in children ages 6 months to 5 years and the safety of mRNA COVID booster doses in people 5+ years (ACIP, 2022f). VAERS or VSD had no evidence of a higher risk of myocarditis in children aged 6 months to 5 years following their primary series. Data did show an increased risk of myocarditis following a first booster dose with a mRNA vaccine in people aged 5+, particularly among male adolescents and young adults. There were 131 reports of myocarditis in individuals aged 5+ after over 123 million booster doses. This safety signal was not significant for individuals aged 5–11. VAERS reports of myocarditis were lower after the first booster than after dose 2 of the primary series. In contrast, VSD found similar rates but with small case numbers, leading to wide confidence intervals and uncertainty. ACIP voted to recommend the Pfizer-BioNTech bivalent booster at a dose of 30 micrograms for individuals ≥12 years and Moderna bivalent booster at a dose of 50 micrograms in people ≥18 years.

TABLE D-2 Continued

Meeting Date	Summary
October 21, 2022	VST provided an update on vaccine safety, which included myocarditis (ACIP, 2022h). Multiple monitoring systems continued to provide evidence of increased myocarditis risk among male adolescents and young adults within a few days following dose 2, including the VAERS, VSD, and Department of Defense systems. FDA data did not show a significant variation in risk between the Pfizer-BioNTech and Moderna vaccines. The VA system reported few cases of myocarditis, likely due to its older patient population. Canada, Israel, and other European countries were reporting similar findings regarding myocarditis risk. Canada and select countries in Northern Europe were observing greater myocarditis risk for the Moderna compared to the Pfizer-BioNTech vaccine. The VaST assessment found a slightly higher risk of myocarditis in men aged 18–29 after the Moderna primary series compared to the Pfizer-BioNTech series and highlighted the limited data available on myocarditis risk following Moderna booster doses.

NOTES: This list was generated based on ACIP documentation archived on the CDC Stacks website and may not include information that was not preserved in the archive. ACIP = Advisory Committee on Immunization Practices; AE = adverse event; CDC = Centers for Disease Control and Prevention; FDA = Food and Drug Administration; RCA = rapid-cycle analysis; VA = Department of Veterans Affairs; VAERS = Vaccine Adverse Event Reporting System; VaST = Vaccine Safety Technical Work group; VSD = Vaccine Safety Datalink; VST = Vaccine Safety Team.

who filed a VAERS report between January 12, 2021, and November 5, 2021. Data collection occurred between August 24, 2021, and January 12, 2022. The study methodology included a two-component survey completed at least 90 days after myocarditis symptoms began. One component was completed by the patient or their guardian and the other by their HCP.

The study followed 519 patients (Kracalik et al., 2022). The median age was 17 years, and 88 percent were male. HCPs indicated that the majority (81 percent) were considered recovered, though 26 percent remained on daily medication related to myocarditis. Some patients reported ongoing issues, including depression (46 percent) and pain (30 percent), but overall quality-of-life scores were similar to prepandemic levels. Most cardiac diagnostic tests showed improvement, with a high percentage of patients returning to normal or baseline values. While 54 percent of follow-up cardiac MRIs showed abnormalities, only 13 percent had findings consistent with active myocarditis, and 68 percent were cleared for full physical activity.

ACIP received updates from VST on the follow-up study. Updates on enrollment and data collection were provided at the October 21, 2021, meeting (Shimabukuro and ACIP, 2021). Preliminary data were reported at the February 4, 2022, meeting (Kracalik, 2022). ACIP was provided preliminary data specifically regarding patients aged 5–17 at the June 23, 2022, meeting (Shimabukuro, 2022e). The results of the HCP survey were presented at the July 19, 2022 meeting (Shimabukuro, 2022d). Final results were published in *The Lancet* in September 2022 (Kracalik et al., 2022). CDC also launched a webpage about the study in August 2021, including how people would be contacted to participate in the study and how the information would be used (NCIRD, 2021d).

Public Interest and Vaccine Confidence

ISO receives vaccine safety questions from HCPs, public health officials, and the public through multiple communication channels (Miller et al., 2023). Between December 1, 2020, and August 31, 2022, ISO received 1,655 inquiries about COVID vaccine safety; myocarditis was the second most common concern, accounting for 9 percent of inquiries. Inquiries on myocarditis were most commonly made by HCPs about the risk following vaccination across age cohorts and CDC's benefit–risk assessment of myocarditis following vaccinations. Inquiries from the public were commonly requesting medical advice for treating myocarditis following vaccination.

CDC regularly published *State of Vaccine Confidence Insights Reports* throughout the COVID PHE, analyzing factors affecting U.S. vaccine uptake and hesitancy. These reports drew data from social media, web searches, media inquiries, polls, and scientific literature. The first report, covering January 24–February 6, 2021, was released on February 12, 2021. Myocarditis was first mentioned in a special report on June 14, 2021, following the authorization and recommendation of the Pfizer-BioNTech vaccine for adolescents aged 12–15. The report highlighted a surge in discussions on social and news media regarding COVID vaccination and myocarditis in adolescents. Parents raised concerns about vaccine safety, the risk of myocarditis compared to its general prevalence, its severity and long-term effects, and whether to proceed with the second dose. Myocarditis remained a recurring topic in these reports throughout the PHE as a factor influencing vaccine confidence and hesitancy, particularly for mRNA COVID vaccines for children and adults (CDC, 2021f,g,h,i, 2022a,b,c,e,f,g, 2023a).

TINNITUS CASE STUDY

Tinnitus is defined as "the perception of sound without an external source" (Tunkel et al., 2014). It is estimated that about one-quarter of the U.S. population experiences tinnitus at any given point in time. People with tinnitus often describe hearing ringing, buzzing, or clicking, among other sounds, in one or both ears. It can be idiopathic, be associated with sensorineural hearing loss, or result from another system disorder, such as cochlear or vascular abnormalities. It is most prevalent in individuals with loud noise exposure. It can significantly impact quality of life and may result in insomnia, depression, or anxiety, among other psychiatric conditions.

Tinnitus was not reported as a postvaccination event for BNT162b2 (Pfizer-BioNTech) or mRNA-1273 (Moderna) in the U.S. clinical trial data used for initial EUA (Baden et al., 2021; Polack et al., 2020). It was reported in the clinical trial data for Ad26.COV2.S (Janssen) (Sadoff et al., 2021). It occurred in six participants in the vaccine group (out of 3,356 participants in the safety subpopulation) compared to zero participants in the placebo group. As a result, Janssen indicated that tinnitus would undergo postmarketing monitoring (Sadoff et al., 2021). Tinnitus was not designated as an AESI warranting proactive monitoring via the U.S. COVID vaccine safety monitoring systems (Gee et al., 2024). It has been reported with other vaccines, including the hepatitis, rabies, measles, and H1N1 vaccines (Harpaz et al., 2022).

Timeline of Events

VaST first reviewed tinnitus and hearing loss associated with COVID vaccines on November 14, 2022 (Markowitz et al., 2024) in response to public interest and concerns following reports of tinnitus in the Janssen vaccine trial. It reviewed data from VAERS and VSD. Reports of tinnitus were rare following Pfizer-BioNTech and Moderna vaccines, with 21.6 and 22.7 cases per million doses administered, respectively. The VSD analysis estimated an incidence of tinnitus per 10,000 person-years of 78, 107, and 85 following the Pfizer-BioNTech, Moderna, and Janssen vaccines, respectively, based on 140 days of follow-up after vaccination. These observed rates were all below the expected background incidence (approximately 116 cases per 10,000 person-years among the general population). VaST determined that, based on the data reviewed through the April 2023 meeting, no safety concerns were identified. Based on a review of summary minutes from public meetings available via the CDC archives website, tinnitus was not included in any VaST assessments presented to ACIP during the PHE.

In 2024, ISO participated in publication of a peer-reviewed study of tinnitus following COVID vaccine (Yih et al., 2024). The study used data from VAERS and VSD and showed no disproportionate reporting of tinnitus in either monitoring system for any vaccine using similar methods to those that had identified the myocarditis safety signal. Although the study did not find strong evidence of increased risk, researchers acknowledged limitations in adjusting for confounding factors, meaning a definitive conclusion could not be reached.

Public Interest and Vaccine Confidence

Between December 2020 and August 2022, approximately 2 percent ($n = 28$) of 1,655 inquiries about COVID vaccine safety received by ISO were about tinnitus (Miller et al., 2023). It made one appearance in the CDC *State of Vaccine Confidence Insights Reports*. Tinnitus It was identified as a new and emerging theme that may be affecting vaccine confidence in the June 10, 2022, edition reflecting the March 14–April 4, 2022, time frame. A World Health Organization Pharmaceuticals newsletter had recently highlighted that the Uppsala Monitoring Centre observed tinnitus after COVID vaccination frequently enough to merit further study (CDC, 2022h). There were 367 reported cases of post-vaccination tinnitus across 10 countries as of February 22, 2022 linked to the Pfizer/BioNTech, Moderna, and AstraZeneca vaccines (CDC, 2022h; WHO, 2022).

MENSTRUAL IRREGULARITIES CASE STUDY

Menstrual irregularities refer to disruptions in the menstrual cycle (NIH, 2017a) and affect approximately 14–25 percent of women (Whitaker and Critchley, 2016). The most common include missed or infrequent periods, heavy or prolonged bleeding, or severe cramps (NIH, 2017b). Menstruation is controlled by a complex balance of hormones, inflammation, and tissue changes (Wong et al., 2022). Since COVID vaccines can cause temporary inflammation, it is biologically plausible that they could briefly disrupt the menstrual cycle and trigger unexpected bleeding.

Menstrual irregularities were not identified as a postvaccination occurrence in the clinical trial data for the Pfizer-BioNTech, Moderna, or Janssen vaccines that supported their initial EUA (Baden et al., 2021; Polack et al., 2020; Sadoff et al., 2021). While vaccination during pregnancy and pregnancy outcomes were AESIs, menstrual irregularities was not predetermined to be an AE warranting proactive safety monitoring (Polack et al., 2020).

Timeline of Events

Reports of menstrual irregularities following COVID vaccination emerged in 2021 via social media and in the news (NIH, n.d.a). VaST reported reviewing outcomes related to menstrual irregularities or vaginal bleeding (Markowitz et al., 2024). The data reviewed were published as an observational cohort study in August 2022 (Markowitz et al., 2024; Wong et al., 2022) that identified 63,815 reports of menstrual irregularities or vaginal bleeding from 62,679 female respondents in V-safe from December 14, 2020 to January 9, 2022. These reports represented 1 percent of all female respondents ≥18 years in V-safe. Menstruation timing (83.6 percent) and menstrual system severity (67 percent) were most commonly reported.

A review of summary minutes from public meetings available on the CDC archives website found no mention of menstrual irregularities in any VaST assessments presented to ACIP during the PHE. During the ACIP meeting on September 1, 2022, menstrual irregularities was identified as a pregnancy and reproductive health outcome being monitored following COVID vaccination in the presentation by VST (Shimabukuro, 2022c); the slides did not include any additional information on menstrual irregularities.

CDC did release information to the public on its website about the impact of COVID vaccination on menstruation and reproductive health in 2021 and 2022 (NCIRD, 2021g, 2022a,b). The "Myths and Facts about COVID-19 Vaccines" webpage addressed the question, "Can being near someone who received a COVID-19 vaccine affect my menstrual cycle?" (NCIRD, 2021g) The "COVID-19 Vaccines for People Who Would Like to Have a Baby" webpage discussed the limited research on the impact of vaccination on the menstrual cycle, noting that while minor, temporary changes—such as variations in cycle length, intervals, and heavier bleeding—had been observed, no evidence suggested it affected fertility (NCIRD, 2022a). The "Frequently Asked Questions about COVID-19 Vaccination" webpage also answered the question, "Do COVID-19 vaccines affect your menstrual cycle?" (NCIRD, 2022b).

In May 2021, the National Institutes of Health (NIH) announced funding for research studies exploring potential links between the COVID vaccine and menstruation (NIH, n.d.b). In August of the same year, NIH announced the five institutions that received funding (NIH, 2021). Research published to date from this funding has found a link between COVID vaccination and small, temporary menstrual changes (Edelman et al., 2022; Ramaiyer et al., 2024). Two studies found an increase in menstrual cycle length (Edelman et al., 2022; Wesselink et al., 2023). A third study found a small increase in menses length (Ramaiyer et al., 2024).

Public Interest and Vaccine Confidence

About 1 percent of 1,666 COVID vaccine safety inquiries made to ISO between December 2020 and August 2022 were related to irregular menses (Miller et al., 2023). Menstrual irregularities first appeared in the CDC *State of Vaccine Confidence Insights Report* on April 28, 2021 (CDC, 2021c). Report #6 stated reports of "atypical menstruation" from women following COVID vaccination had "been co-opted and incorporated into misinformation narratives that warn of a link between COVID-19 vaccination and infertility." Multiple reports in May 2021 highlighted growing concerns about the impact of COVID vaccination on menstrual cycles and social media, including "viral shedding," whereby the menstrual cycle of unvaccinated individuals could be influenced through exposure to vaccinated individuals (CDC, 2021d,e). The *State of Vaccine Confidence Insight Reports* consistently highlighted consumer concerns about menstrual changes, potential effects on fertility, and likely impact on vaccine hesitancy through mid-2022 (CDC, 2021g,i, 2022b,c,d, 2023a).

CHIKUNGUNYA VACCINE CASE STUDY

Chikungunya is a viral illness transmitted by mosquitoes (WHO, 2025). It was first detected in Tanzania in 1952 and later identified in various countries across Africa and Asia. Since 2024, outbreaks have become more frequent and widespread, largely due to viral mutations that have enhanced its ability to spread through *Aedes albopictus* mosquitoes. The disease has now been documented in 110 nations across Africa, Asia, Europe, and the Americas. It typically begins with a sudden fever, often accompanied by joint pain that can be debilitating. Although it is rarely fatal, some cases involve eye, heart, and neurological complications.

Between 2006 and 2013, an average of 28 U.S. cases per year were identified (WHO, 2025). The first local transmission in the Americas was recorded in the Caribbean in late 2013, leading to subsequent cases in the United States. It became a nationally notifiable disease in 2015. In 2024, 199 U.S. cases were reported, all travel associated; no locally acquired cases have been reported since 2019.

On November 9, 2023, FDA approved a live, attenuated vaccine (CHIK-LA) "for the prevention of disease caused by chikungunya virus in individuals 18 years of age and older who are at increased risk of exposure to chikungunya virus" under statutory provisions and regulations for accelerated approval (Kaslow, 2023). On February 28, 2024, ACIP recommended it "for persons aged $\geq$18 years traveling to a country or territory where there is a chikungunya outbreak" and "laboratory workers with potential for exposure to chikungunya virus" (ACIP, 2024). CHIK-LA vaccine is administered intramuscularly as a single dose (CDC, 2025b). Headache, fatigue, myalgia, arthralgia, injection-site pain, pyrexia, and nausea occurred in $\geq$10 percent of clinical trial participants (Schneider et al., 2023). Serious AEs identified during the Phase 3 clinical trial of adults were infections and infestations (0.3 percent of intervention participants); injury, poisoning, and procedural complications (0.3 percent); psychiatric disorders (0.2 percent); and cardiac disorders (0.2 percent). The vaccine package insert contains a warning for severe or prolonged chikungunya-like adverse reactions (FDA, n.d.).

Timeline of Events

In February 2025, CDC reported that five individuals aged 65+ were hospitalized with cardiac or neurological symptoms after recently receiving CHIK-LA vaccine (Howard, 2025; Twenter, 2025). On February 25, 2025, CDC posted an update to its webpage on the vaccine for HCPs (CDC, 2025b; Howard, 2025): "CDC is currently investigating five hospitalizations for cardiac or neurologic events following vaccination with [CHIK-LA] among people 65 years of age and older. This topic will be discussed at an upcoming meeting of ACIP. Health care providers should discuss the benefits and risks of vaccination with individual travelers based on their age, destination, trip duration, and planned activities."

The ACIP meeting scheduled for February 26–28, 2025, was postponed "to accommodate public comment in advance of the meeting." The rescheduled meeting occurred on April 15–16, 2025 (CDC, 2025a) and included a presentation on postlicensure surveillance for AEs following CHIK-LA based on data from VAERS by the Chikungunya Vaccines Work Group (Hills, 2025). VAERS had 28 AE reports from May through December 2024, including 22 nonserious and six serious events. Among the serious AEs, five resulted in hospitalization and one was an "other medically important event."

The presentation included deidentified case summaries of the six serious AEs reported to VAERS (Hills, 2025), which all involved men aged 67–86 with comorbidities. All received CHIK-LA vaccine for upcoming travel. Three had received coadministered vaccines, either the inactive Japanese encephalitis or oral, live typhoid vaccines. Symptom onset began within 3–5 days following vaccine administration. Among the five individuals who were hospitalized, three were discharged with encephalopathy diagnoses, one with aseptic meningitis, and one with atrial flutter and non-ST segment elevation myocardial infarction. The sixth individual was not hospitalized but was diagnosed with worsened and prolonged hypotension with preexisting cardiomyopathy and hypotension by an internist.

The presentation described how the Clinical Immunization Safety Assessment (CISA) Project was consulted (Hills, 2025). For each report, at least one CISA expert assessed association of the serious AE and CHIK-LA vaccine. Several factors supported possible causality: events began 3–5 days after vaccination; association with other vaccines was less likely for the three patients with coadministration; clear alternate etiologies were not identified; discharge summaries of the five hospitalized patients noted potential association with vaccination; and laboratory testing resulted suggested an association with CHIK-LA vaccine for two patients.

The presentation also described how VAERS reports and IQVIA data were used to calculate risk estimates for serious AEs and hospitalizations among persons 65+ (Hills, 2025). The analysis yielded an estimated rate of serious AEs of 82 per 100,000 doses or one serious AE per 1,220 doses and an estimated rate of hospitalization of 68 per 100,000 doses or one hospitalization per 1,471 doses.

The Chikungunya Vaccine Work Group's assessment that being age 65+ should be a precaution for CHIK-LA vaccine (Hills, 2025). It proposed revising the ACIP recommendations for the use of the vaccine among travelers—specifically, by removing adults over 65 from the group for whom the vaccine may be considered when traveling to areas with chikungunya transmission within the last 5 years but no current outbreak. ACIP voted to accept this change to the chikungunya vaccine recommendations (BroadcastCDC, 2025).

REFERENCES

ACIP (Advisory Committee on Immunization Practices). 2021a. *Meeting of the Advisory Committee on Immunization Practices (ACIP), August 30, 2021, Summary Minutes.* https://stacks.cdc.gov/view/cdc/157586 (accessed June 4, 2025).

ACIP. 2021b. *Meeting of the Advisory Committee on Immunization Practices (ACIP), June 23, 2021, Summary Minutes.* https://stacks.cdc.gov/view/cdc/157583 (accessed June 4, 2025).

ACIP. 2021c. *Meeting of the Advisory Committee on Immunization Practices (ACIP), September 22-23, 2021 Summary Minutes.* https://stacks.cdc.gov/view/cdc/114944 (accessed June 4, 2025).

ACIP. 2022a. *Meeting of the Advisory Committee on Immunization Practices (ACIP), April 20, 2022 Summary Minutes.* https://stacks.cdc.gov/view/cdc/122387 (accessed June 4, 2025).

ACIP. 2022b. *Meeting of the Advisory Committee on Immunization Practices (ACIP), January 5, 2022 Summary Minutes.* https://stacks.cdc.gov/view/cdc/122251 (accessed June 4, 2025).

ACIP. 2022c. *Meeting of the Advisory Committee on Immunization Practices (ACIP), July 19, 2022, Executive Summary.* https://stacks.cdc.gov/view/cdc/122557 (accessed June 4, 2025).

ACIP. 2022d. *Meeting of the Advisory Committee on Immunization Practices (ACIP), June 17-18, 2022, Summary Minutes.* https://stacks.cdc.gov/view/cdc/157588 (accessed June 4, 2025).

ACIP. 2022e. *Meeting of the Advisory Committee on Immunization Practices (ACIP), May 19, 2022 Summary Minutes.* https://stacks.cdc.gov/view/cdc/122458 (accessed June 4, 2025).

ACIP. 2022f. *Meeting of the Advisory Committee on Immunization Practices (ACIP), September 1, 2022, Meeting Summary.* https://stacks.cdc.gov/view/cdc/122625 (accessed June 4, 2025).

ACIP. 2022g. *Meeting of the Advisory Committee on Immunization Practices (ACIP), June 22-23, 2022 Summary Minutes.* https://stacks.cdc.gov/view/cdc/122517 (accessed June 4, 2025).

ACIP. 2022h. *Meeting of the Advisory Committee on Immunization Practices (ACIP), October 20-21, 2021 Summary Minutes.* https://stacks.cdc.gov/view/cdc/118729 (accessed June 4, 2025).

ACIP. 2024. *Meeting of the Advisory Committee on Immunization Practices (ACIP).* https://www.cdc.gov/acip/downloads/minutes/summary-2024-02-28-29-508.pdf (accessed June 4, 2025).

Ammirati, E., M. Frigerio, E. D. Adler, C. Basso, D. H. Birnie, M. Brambatti, M. G. Friedrich, K. Klingel, J. Lehtonen, and J. J. Moslehi. 2020. Management of acute myocarditis and chronic inflammatory cardiomyopathy: An expert consensus document. *Circulation: Heart Failure* 13(11):e007405. https://doi.org/10.1161/CIRCHEARTFAILURE.120.007405.

Ammirati, E., and J. J. Moslehi. 2023. Diagnosis and treatment of acute myocarditis: A review. *JAMA* 329(13):1098–1113. https://doi.org/10.1001/jama.2023.3371.

Arness, M. K., R. E. Eckart, S. S. Love, J. E. Atwood, T. S. Wells, R. J. Engler, L. C. Collins, S. L. Ludwig, J. R. Riddle, and J. D. Grabenstein. 2004. Myopericarditis following smallpox vaccination. *American Journal of Epidemiology* 160(7):642–651.

Baden, L. R., H. M. El Sahly, B. Essink, K. Kotloff, S. Frey, R. Novak, D. Diemert, S. A. Spector, N. Rouphael, and C. B. Creech. 2021. Efficacy and safety of the mRNA-1273 SARS-CoV-2 vaccine. *New England Journal of Medicine* 384(5):403–416. https://doi.org/10.1056/NEJMoa2035389.

Basso, C. 2022. Myocarditis. *New England Journal of Medicine* 387(16):1488–1500. https://doi.org/10.1056/NEJMra2114478.

BroadcastCDC. 2025.*Centers for Disease Control and Prevention (CDC)*. https://www.youtube.com/live/zN4ACg2mEzw (accessed July 8, 2025).

CDC (Centers for Disease Control and Prevention). 2003. Update: Cardiac-related events during the civilian smallpox vaccination program—United States, 2003. *MMWR* 52(21):492–496.

CDC. 2021a. *CDC Expands Eligibility for COVID-19 Booster Shots*. https://stacks.cdc.gov/view/cdc/111902 (accessed June 4, 2025).

CDC. 2021b. *CDC Expands Eligibility for COVID-19 Booster Shots: Media Statement for Immediate Release: Thursday, October 21, 2021*. https://stacks.cdc.gov/view/cdc/110980 (accessed June 4, 2025).

CDC. 2021c. *COVID-19 State of Vaccine Confidence Insights Report report 6*. https://stacks.cdc.gov/view/cdc/153014 (accessed June 4, 2025).

CDC. 2021d. *COVID-19 State of Vaccine Confidence Insights Report report 7*. https://stacks.cdc.gov/view/cdc/153026 (accessed June 4, 2025).

CDC. 2021e. *COVID-19 State of Vaccine Confidence Insights Report report 8*. https://stacks.cdc.gov/view/cdc/153009 (accessed June 4, 2025).

CDC. 2021f. *COVID-19 State of Vaccine Confidence Insights Report report 10*. https://stacks.cdc.gov/view/cdc/153022 (accessed June 4, 2025).

CDC. 2021g. *COVID-19 State of Vaccine Confidence Insights Report report 12*. https://stacks.cdc.gov/view/cdc/142768 (accessed June 4, 2025).

CDC. 2021h. *COVID-19 State of Vaccine Confidence Insights Report report 16*. https://stacks.cdc.gov/view/cdc/142715 (accessed June 4, 2025).

CDC. 2021i. *COVID-19 State of Vaccine Confidence Insights Report report 17*. https://stacks.cdc.gov/view/cdc/142780 (accessed June 4, 2025).

CDC. 2022a. *COVID-19 State of Vaccine Confidence Insights Report report 21*. https://stacks.cdc.gov/view/cdc/153027 (accessed June 4, 2025).

CDC. 2022b. *COVID-19 State of Vaccine Confidence Insights Report report 22*. https://stacks.cdc.gov/view/cdc/152999 (accessed June 4, 2025).

CDC. 2022c. *COVID-19 State of Vaccine Confidence Insights Report report 23*. https://stacks.cdc.gov/view/cdc/152996 (accessed June 4, 2025).

CDC. 2022d. *COVID-19 State of Vaccine Confidence Insights Report report 25*. https://stacks.cdc.gov/view/cdc/142723 (accessed June 4, 2025).

CDC. 2022e. *COVID-19 State of Vaccine Confidence Insights Report report 26*. https://stacks.cdc.gov/view/cdc/142726 (accessed June 4, 2025).

CDC. 2022f. *COVID-19 State of Vaccine Confidence Insights Report: Summary report: COVID-19 vaccines for children*. https://stacks.cdc.gov/view/cdc/114927 (accessed June 4, 2025).

CDC. 2022g. *COVID-19 State of Vaccine Confidence Insights Report; report 25, May 12, 2022.* https://stacks.cdc.gov/view/cdc/117453 (accessed June 4, 2025).

CDC. 2022h. *COVID-19 State of Vaccine Confidence Insights Report; report 26, June 10, 2022.* https://stacks.cdc.gov/view/cdc/118650 (accessed June 4, 2025).

CDC. 2023a. *CDC's COVID-19 State of Vaccine Confidence Insights Report: Quarter 3 report, January 26, 2023.* https://stacks.cdc.gov/view/cdc/124197 (accessed June 4, 2025).

CDC. 2023b. *Clinical considerations: Myocarditis and pericarditis after receipt of COVID-19 vaccines among adolescents and young adults.* https://www.cdc.gov/vaccines/covid-19/clinical-considerations/myocarditis.html (accessed June 4, 2025).

CDC. 2024. *CDC museum COVID-19 timeline.* https://www.cdc.gov/museum/timeline/covid19.html (accessed June 3, 2025).

CDC. 2025a. *ACIP meeting information.* https://www.cdc.gov/acip/meetings/index.html (accessed June 4, 2025).

CDC. 2025b. *Chikungunya Vaccine Information for Healthcare Providers.* https://www.cdc.gov/chikungunya/hcp/vaccine/index.html#cdc_generic_section_3-vaccine-immunogenicity-and-side-effects (accessed June 4, 2025).

Edelman, A., E. R. Boniface, V. Male, S. T. Cameron, E. Benhar, L. Han, K. A. Matteson, A. Van Lamsweerde, J. T. Pearson, and B. G. Darney. 2022. Association between menstrual cycle length and COVID-19 vaccination: Global, retrospective cohort study of prospectively collected data. *BMJ Medicine* 1(1):e000297. https://doi.org/10.1136/bmjmed-2022-000297.

FDA (Food and Drug Administration). n.d. *Highlights of Prescribing Information.* https://www.fda.gov/files/vaccines%2C%20blood%20&%20biologics/published/Package-Insert-IXCHIQ.pdf (accessed June 4, 2025).

Gargano, J. W. 2021. Use of mRNA COVID-19 vaccine after reports of myocarditis among vaccine recipients: Update from the Advisory Committee on Immunization Practices—United States, June 2021. *MMWR* 70. https://doi.org/10.15585/mmwr.mm7027e2.

Gee, J., T. T. Shimabukuro, J. R. Su, D. Shay, M. Ryan, S. V. Basavaraju, K. R. Broder, M. Clark, C. B. Creech, and F. Cunningham. 2024. Overview of U.S. COVID-19 vaccine safety surveillance systems. *Vaccine* 42:125748. https://doi.org/10.1016/j.vaccine.2024.02.065.

Guarino, B., A. Eunjung Cha, J. Wood, and G. Witte. 2020. "The weapon that will end the war": First coronavirus vaccine shots given outside trials in U.S. *The Washington Post*, December 14.

Harpaz, R., W. DuMouchel, R. Van Manen, A. Nip, S. Bright, A. Szarfman, J. Tonning, and M. Lerch. 2022. Signaling COVID-19 vaccine adverse events. *Drug Safety* 45(7):765–780. https://doi.org/10.1007/s40264-022-01186-z.

Hills, S. 2025. *Surveillance for Adverse Events Following Use of Live Attenuated Chikungunya Vaccine and Its Use Among Travelers.* https://www.cdc.gov/acip/downloads/slides-2025-04-15-16/04-Hills-chikungunya-508.pdf (accessed June 4, 2025).

Howard, J. 2025. CDC investgating hospitalizations of five people who recently received chikungunya vaccine. *CNN*, February 27.

Kaslow, D. C. 2023. *Accelerated BLA Approval.* Food and Drug Administration. https://www.fda.gov/media/173759/download?attachment (accessed August 26, 2025).

Klein, N. P. 2021. *Myocarditis Analyses in the Vaccine Safety Datalink: Rapid Cycle Analyses and "Head-to-Head" Product Companies.* https://stacks.cdc.gov/view/cdc/110921 (accessed June 4, 2025).

Klein, N. P. 2022. *Myocarditis Analyses in the Vaccine Safety Datalink: Rapid cycle Analyses and "Head-to-Head" Product Comparisons.* https://stacks.cdc.gov/view/cdc/114163 (accessed July 8, 2025).

Kracalik, I. 2022. *Myocarditis Outcomes Following mRNA COVID-19 Vaccination: Preliminary Data: Data Are Subject to Change.* https://stacks.cdc.gov/view/cdc/114157 (accessed June 4, 2025).

Kracalik, I., M. E. Oster, K. R. Broder, M. M. Cortese, M. Glover, K. Shields, C. B. Creech, B. Romanson, S. Novosad, and J. Soslow. 2022. Outcomes at least 90 days since onset of myocarditis after mRNA COVID-19 vaccination in adolescents and young adults in the USA: A follow-up surveillance study. *Lancet Child & Adolescent Health* 6(11):788–798. https://doi.org/10.1016/S2352-4642(22)00244-9.

Lee, G. M., and R. H. Hopkins. 2021. *COVID-19 Vaccine Safety Technical (VaST) Work Group*. https://stacks.cdc.gov/view/cdc/108330 (accessed June 4, 2025).

Markowitz, L. E., R. H. Hopkins, Jr., K. R. Broder, G. M. Lee, K. M. Edwards, M. F. Daley, L. A. Jackson, J. C. Nelson, L. E. Riley, and V. V. McNally. 2024. COVID-19 Vaccine Safety Technical (VaST) Work Group: Enhancing vaccine safety monitoring during the pandemic. *Vaccine* 42:125549. https://doi.org/10.1016/j.vaccine.2023.12.059.

Mei, R., E. Raschi, E. Forcesi, I. Diemberger, F. De Ponti, and E. Poluzzi. 2018. Myocarditis and pericarditis after immunization: Gaining insights through the Vaccine Adverse Event Reporting System. *International Journal of Cardiology* 273:183–186. https://doi.org/10.1016/j.ijcard.2018.09.054.

Mevorach, D., E. Anis, N. Cedar, M. Bromberg, E. J. Haas, E. Nadir, S. Olsha-Castell, D. Arad, T. Hasin, and N. Levi. 2021. Myocarditis after BNT162B2 mRNA vaccine against COVID-19 in Israel. *New England Journal of Medicine* 385(23):2140–2149. https://doi.org/10.1056/NEJMoa2109730.

Miller, E. R., P. L. Moro, T. T. Shimabukuro, G. Carlock, S. N. Davis, E. M. Freeborn, A. L. Roberts, J. Gee, A. W. Taylor, and R. Gallego. 2023. COVID-19 vaccine safety inquiries to the Centers for Disease Control and Prevention Immunization Safety Office. *Vaccine* 41(27):3960–3963. https://doi.org/10.1016/j.vaccine.2023.05.054.

Montgomery, J., M. Ryan, R. Engler, D. Hoffman, B. McClenathan, L. Collins, D. Loran, D. Hrncir, K. Herring, and M. Platzer. 2021. Myocarditis following immunization with mRNA COVID-19 vaccines in members of the U.S. military. *JAMA Cardiology* 6(10):1202–1206. https://doi.org/10.1001/jamacardio.2021.2833.

Nagai, T., T. Inomata, T. Kohno, T. Sato, A. Tada, T. Kubo, K. Nakamura, N. Oyama-Manabe, Y. Ikeda, and T. Fujino. 2023. JCS 2023 guideline on the diagnosis and treatment of myocarditis. *Circulation Journal* 87(5):674–754. https://doi.org/10.1253/circj.CJ-22-0696.

NCIRD (National Center for Immunization and Respiratory Diseases). 2021a. *COVID-19 VaST Work Group Report—May 17, 2021*. https://archive.cdc.gov/www_cdc_gov/vaccines/acip/work-groups-vast/report-2021-05-17.html (accessed June 4, 2025).

NCIRD. 2021b. *COVID-19 Vaccines That Require 2 Shots*. https://stacks.cdc.gov/view/cdc/106798 (accessed June 4, 2025).

NCIRD. 2021c. *COVID-19 VaST Work Group Report—May 24, 2021*. https://archive.cdc.gov/www_cdc_gov/vaccines/acip/work-groups-vast/report-2021-05-24.html (accessed June 4, 2025).

NCIRD. 2021d. *Investigation of Long-Term Effects of Myocarditis After mRNA COVID-19 Vaccination*. https://stacks.cdc.gov/view/cdc/109084 (accessed June 4, 2025).

NCIRD. 2021e. *Moderna COVID-19 Vaccine Overview and Safety*. https://stacks.cdc.gov/view/cdc/109018 (accessed June 4, 2025).

NCIRD. 2021f. *Myocarditis and Pericarditis Following mRNA COVID-19 Vaccination*. https://stacks.cdc.gov/view/cdc/106641 (accessed June 4, 2025).

NCIRD. 2021g. *Myths and Facts About COVID-19 Vaccines*. https://stacks.cdc.gov/view/cdc/108736 (accessed June 4, 2025).

NCIRD. 2021h. *Pfizer-BioNTech COVID-19 Vaccine Overview and Safety*. https://stacks.cdc.gov/view/cdc/107502 (accessed June 4, 2025).

NCIRD. 2021i. *Selected Adverse Events Reported After COVID-19 Vaccination*. https://stacks.cdc.gov/view/cdc/107048 (accessed June 4, 2025).

NCIRD. 2022a. *COVID-19 Vaccines for People Who Would Like to Have a Baby*. https://stacks.cdc.gov/view/cdc/115013 (accessed August 25, 2025).

NCIRD. 2022b. *Frequently Asked Questions About COVID-19 Vaccination.* https://stacks.cdc.gov/view/cdc/116238 (accessed June 4, 2025).

NIH (National Institutes of Health). n.d.a. *COVID-19 Vaccines and Menstruation.* https://www.nichd.nih.gov/research/supported/COVID/NICHD_Populations/COVID-Vaccines_Menstruation (accessed June 4, 2025).

NIH. n.d.b. *Notice of Special Interest (NOSI) to Encourage Administrative Supplement Applications to Investigate COVID-19 Vaccination and Menstruation (admin supp clinical trial optional).* https://grants.nih.gov/grants/guide/notice-files/NOT-HD-21-035.html (accessed June 4, 2025).

NIH. 2017a. *Menstruation and Menstrual Problems.* https://www.nichd.nih.gov/health/topics/menstruation (accessed June 4, 2025).

NIH. 2017b. *What Are Menstrual Irregularities?* https://www.nichd.nih.gov/health/topics/menstruation/conditioninfo/irregularities#f2 (accessed June 4, 2025).

NIH. 2021. *Item of Interest: NIH Funds Studies to Assess Potential Effects of COVID-19 Vaccination on Menstruation.* https://www.nichd.nih.gov/newsroom/news/083021-COVID-19-vaccination-menstruation (accessed June 4, 2025).

Oliver, S. E. 2021. *ETR framework: Pfizer-BioNTech COVID-19 Vaccine in Children Aged 5–11 Years.* https://stacks.cdc.gov/view/cdc/111212 (accessed June 4, 2025).

Oster, M. E. 2021a. *mRNA COVID-19 Vaccine-Associated Myocarditis.* https://stacks.cdc.gov/view/cdc/111208 (accessed June 4, 2021).

Oster, M. E. 2021b. *Overview of Myocarditis and Pericarditis.* https://stacks.cdc.gov/view/cdc/108328 (accessed June 4, 2025).

Polack, F. P., S. J. Thomas, N. Kitchin, J. Absalon, A. Gurtman, S. Lockhart, J. L. Perez, G. Pérez Marc, E. D. Moreira, and C. Zerbini. 2020. Safety and efficacy of the BNT162b2 mRNA COVID-19 vaccine. *New England Journal of Medicine* 383(27):2603–2615. https://doi.org/10.1056/NEJMoa2034577.

Poland, G. A., J. D. Grabenstein, and J. M. Neff. 2005. The U.S. smallpox vaccination program: A review of a large modern era smallpox vaccination implementation program. *Vaccine* 23(17–18):2078–2081. https://doi.org/10.1016/j.vaccine.2005.01.012.

Ramaiyer, M., M. El Sabeh, J. Zhu, A. Shea, D. Segev, G. Yenokyan, and M. A. Borahay. 2024. The association of COVID-19 vaccination and menstrual health: A period-tracking app-based cohort study. *Vaccine: X* 19:100501. https://doi.org/10.1016/j.jvacx.2024.100501.

Sadoff, J., G. Gray, A. Vandebosch, V. Cárdenas, G. Shukarev, B. Grinsztejn, P. A. Goepfert, C. Truyers, H. Fennema, and B. Spiessens. 2021. Safety and efficacy of single-dose Ad26.COV2.S vaccine against COVID-19. *New England Journal of Medicine* 384(23):2187–2201. https://doi.org/10.1056/NEJMoa2101544.

Schneider, M., M. Narciso-Abraham, S. Hadl, R. McMahon, S. Toepfer, U. Fuchs, R. Hochreiter, A. Bitzer, K. Kosulin, and J. Larcher-Senn. 2023. Safety and immunogenicity of a single-shot live-attenuated chikungunya vaccine: A double-blind, multicentre, randomised, placebo-controlled, Phase 3 trial. *Lancet* 401(10394):2138–2147. https://doi.org/10.1016/S0140-6736(23)00641-4.

Shimabukuro, T. 2022a. *COVID-19 Vaccine Safety Updates: Primary Series in Children Ages 5–11 Years.* https://stacks.cdc.gov/view/cdc/117469 (accessed June 4, 2025).

Shimabukuro, T. 2022b. *Updates on Myocarditis and Pericarditis Following Moderna COVID-19 Vaccination.* https://stacks.cdc.gov/view/cdc/114156 (accessed June 4, 2025).

Shimabukuro, T. T. 2021a. *COVID-19 Vaccine Booster Dose Safety.* https://stacks.cdc.gov/view/cdc/111887#you-contain (accessed June 4, 2025).

Shimabukuro, T. T. 2021b. *COVID-19 Vaccine Safety Monitoring in Children.* https://stacks.cdc.gov/view/cdc/111209 (accessed June 4, 2025).

Shimabukuro, T. T. 2021c. *COVID-19 Vaccine Safety Updates.* https://stacks.cdc.gov/view/cdc/105736 (accessed June 3, 2025).

Shimabukuro, T. T. 2021d. *COVID-19 Vaccine Safety Updates.* https://stacks.cdc.gov/view/cdc/108329 (accessed June 4, 2025).
Shimabukuro, T. T. 2022c. *COVID-19 Vaccine Safety Update: Primary Series in Young Children and Booster Doses in Older Children and Adults.* https://stacks.cdc.gov/view/cdc/120824 (accessed June 4, 2025).
Shimabukuro, T. T. 2022d. *Myocarditis Following mRNA COVID-19 Vaccination.* https://stacks.cdc.gov/view/cdc/119451 (accessed June 4, 2025).
Shimabukuro, T. T. 2022e. *Update on Myocarditis Following mRNA COVID-19 Vaccination.* https://stacks.cdc.gov/view/cdc/118585 (accessed June 4, 2025).
Shimabukuro, T., and ACIP (Advisory Committee on Immunization Practices). 2021. COVID-19 vaccine safety updates. 2021. Paper read at ACIP Meeting on COVID-19 Vaccines, October 21.
Su, J. R. 2021a. *Adverse Events Among Children Ages 5–11 Years After COVID-19 Vaccination: Updates from V-Safe and the Vaccine Adverse Event Reporting System (VAERS).* https://stacks.cdc.gov/View/cdc/112668 (accessed June 4, 2025).
Su, J. R. 2021b. *Myopericarditis following COVID-19 vaccination: Updates from the Vaccine Adverse Event Reporting System (VAERS).* https://stacks.cdc.gov/view/cdc/110920 (accessed June 4, 2025).
Talbot, H. K., and R. H. Hopkins. 2021. *COVID-19 Vaccine Safety Technical (VaST) Work Group.* https://stacks.cdc.gov/view/cdc/110922 (accessed June 4, 2025).
Talbot, H. K., and R. H. Hopkins, Jr. 2022a. *COVID-19 Vaccine Safety Technical (VaST) Work Group Safety Assessment.* https://stacks.cdc.gov/view/cdc/114158 (accessed June 4, 2025).
Talbot, H. K., and R. H. Hopkins, Jr. 2022b. *COVID-19 Vaccines Safety Technical (VaST) Work Group: VaST Assessment.* https://stacks.cdc.gov/view/cdc/117470 (accessed June 4, 2025).
Talbot, H. K., and R. H. Hopkins. 2022c. *COVID-19 Vaccine Safety Technical (VaST) Work Group Safety Assessment.* https://stacks.cdc.gov/view/cdc/111888 (accessed June 4, 2025).
Tunkel, D. E., C. A. Bauer, G. H. Sun, R. M. Rosenfeld, S. S. Chandrasekhar, E. R. Cunningham Jr, S. M. Archer, B. W. Blakley, J. M. Carter, and E. C. Granieri. 2014. Clinical practice guideline: Tinnitus. *Otolaryngology—Head and Neck Surgery* 151(2_suppl):S1–S40. https://doi.org/10.1177/0194599814545323.
Twenter, P. 2025. *CDC Probes Hospitalizations After Chikungunya Vaccination.* https://www.beckershospitalreview.com/public-health/cdc-probes-hospitalizations-after-chikungunya-vaccination/ (accessed June 4, 2025).
VAERS (Vaccine Adverse Event Reporting System). n.d. *Vaccine Adverse Event Reporting System.* https://vaers.hhs.gov/ (accessed June 3, 2025).
Wallace, M., and S. E. Oliver. 2021. *COVID-19 mRNA vaccines in adolescents and young adults: Benefit-risk discussion.* https://stacks.cdc.gov/view/cdc/108331 (accessed June 4, 2025).
Wesselink, A. K., S. M. Lovett, J. Weinberg, R. J. Geller, T. R. Wang, A. K. Regan, M. D. Willis, R. B. Perkins, J. J. Yland, and M. R. Koenig. 2023. COVID-19 vaccination and menstrual cycle characteristics: A prospective cohort study. *Vaccine* 41(29):4327–4334. https://doi.org/10.1016/j.vaccine.2023.06.012.
Whitaker, L., and H. O. Critchley. 2016. Abnormal uterine bleeding. *Best Practice & Research Clinical Obstetrics & Gynaecology* 34:54–65. https://doi.org/10.1016/j.bpobgyn.2015.11.012.
WHO (World Health Organization). 2022. *WHO Pharmaceuticals Newsletter No. 1 2022.* https://iris.who.int/bitstream/handle/10665/351326/9789240042452-eng.pdf?sequence=1&isAllowed=y (accessed June 4, 2025).

WHO. 2025. *Chikungunya.* https://www.who.int/news-room/fact-sheets/detail/chikungunya (accessed June 4, 2025).
Wong, K. K., C. M. Heilig, A. Hause, T. R. Myers, C. K. Olson, J. Gee, P. Marquez, P. Strid, and D. K. Shay. 2022. Menstrual irregularities and vaginal bleeding after COVID-19 vaccination reported to V-Safe active surveillance, USA in December, 2020–January, 2022: An observational cohort study. *Lancet Digital Health* 4(9):e667–e675. https://doi.org/10.1016/S2589-7500(22)00125-X.
Woodworth, K. R. 2021. *Interim Clinical Considerations for COVID-19 Vaccine in Children Ages 5–11 Years.* https://stacks.cdc.gov/view/cdc/111211 (accessed June 4, 2025).
Yih, W. K., J. Duffy, J. R. Su, S. Bazel, B. Fireman, L. Hurley, J. C. Maro, P. Marquez, P. Moro, and N. Nair. 2024. Tinnitus after COVID-19 vaccination: Findings from the Vaccine Adverse Event Reporting System and the Vaccine Safety Datalink. *American Journal of Otolaryngology* 45(6):104448. https://doi.org/10.1016/j.amjoto.2024.104448.

Appendix E

Catalog of Data-Driven Literature from CDC Vaccine Safety Monitoring

This catalog presents a curated summary of peer-reviewed, data-driven studies supported by the CDC Immunization Safety Office (ISO) during the COVID public health emergency (PHE). These studies move beyond descriptive reporting to apply structured analytical methods—such as cohort comparisons, rapid-cycle analyses, and signal detection algorithms—to evaluate the safety of authorized COVID vaccines. They leverage surveillance systems, including the Vaccine Adverse Event Reporting System (VAERS), Vaccine Safety Datalink (VSD), and V-safe, and draw on electronic health record data, immunization registries, and patient self-reporting tools.

Grouped thematically, each summary highlights the analytic focus of the study, including the population studied, surveillance systems used, and major insights about vaccine safety during the public health response.

GENERAL SAFETY SURVEILLANCE AND SIGNAL DETECTION

- **A Broad Assessment of COVID-19 Vaccine Safety Using Tree-Based Data Mining in the Vaccine Safety Datalink (Yih et al., 2023a)**
Data-driven analysis of adverse events (AEs) following COVID vaccination using surveillance systems.

Included a range of adult and pediatric populations, applying broad surveillance to detect and characterize trends in AE reporting and signal strength.

- **A Safety Study Evaluating Non-COVID-19 Mortality Risk Following COVID-19 Vaccination (Xu et al., 2023)**

  Data-driven analysis of AEs following COVID vaccination using surveillance systems.

  Included a range of adult and pediatric populations, applying broad surveillance to detect and characterize trends in AE reporting and signal strength.

- **Anxiety-Related Adverse Event Clusters After Janssen COVID-19—Five U.S. Mass Vaccination Sites, April 2021 (Hause, 2021a)**

  Data-driven analysis of AEs following COVID vaccination using surveillance systems.

  Included a range of adult and pediatric populations, applying broad surveillance to detect and characterize trends in AE reporting and signal strength.

- **Association Between History of SARS-CoV-2 Infection and Severe Systemic Adverse Events After mRNA COVID-19 Vaccination Among U.S. Adults (Tompkins et al., 2022)**

  Data-driven analysis of AEs following COVID vaccination using surveillance systems.

  Included a range of adult and pediatric populations, applying broad surveillance to detect and characterize trends in AE reporting and signal strength.

- **Case Series of Thrombosis With Thrombocytopenia Syndrome After COVID-19 Vaccination—United States, December 2020 to August 2021 (See et al., 2022)**

  Data-driven analysis of AEs following COVID vaccination using surveillance systems.

  Included a range of adult and pediatric populations, applying broad surveillance to detect and characterize trends in AE reporting and signal strength.

- **COVID-19 Vaccination and Non-COVID-19 Mortality Risk—Seven Integrated Health Care Organizations, United States, December 14, 2020–July 31, 2021 (Xu et al., 2021)**

  Data-driven analysis of AEs following COVID vaccination using surveillance systems.

  Included a range of adult and pediatric populations, applying broad surveillance to detect and characterize trends in AE reporting and signal strength.

- **First Month of COVID-19 Vaccine Safety Monitoring—United States, December 14, 2020–January 13, 2021 (Gee et al., 2021)**
  Summaries of real-world AE reporting and surveillance outcomes for COVID vaccines.
  Included a range of adult and pediatric populations, applying broad surveillance to detect and characterize trends in AE reporting and signal strength.

- **Guillain-Barré Syndrome After COVID-19 Vaccination in the Vaccine Safety Datalink (Hanson et al., 2021)**
  Data-driven analysis of AEs following COVID vaccination using surveillance systems.
  Included a range of adult and pediatric populations, applying broad surveillance to detect and characterize trends in AE reporting and signal strength.

- **Incidence of Guillain-Barré Syndrome After COVID-19 Vaccination in the Vaccine Safety Datalink (Hanson et al., 2022)**
  Data-driven analysis of AEs following COVID vaccination using surveillance systems.
  Included a range of adult and pediatric populations, applying broad surveillance to detect and characterize trends in AE reporting and signal strength.

- **Menstrual Irregularities and Vaginal Bleeding After COVID-19 Vaccination Reported to V-safe Active Surveillance, USA in December, 2020–January, 2022: An Observational Cohort Study (Wong et al., 2022)**
  Data-driven analysis of AEs following COVID vaccination using surveillance systems.
  Included a range of adult and pediatric populations, applying broad surveillance to detect and characterize trends in AE reporting and signal strength.

- **Mortality Risk After COVID-19 Vaccination: A Self-Controlled Case Series Study (Xu et al., 2024)**
  Data-driven analysis of AEs following COVID vaccination using surveillance systems.
  Included a range of adult and pediatric populations, applying broad surveillance to detect and characterize trends in AE reporting and signal strength.

- **Notes from the Field: Safety Monitoring of Novavax COVID-19 Vaccine Among Persons Aged ≥12 Years—United States, July 13, 2022–March 13, 2023 (Romanson et al., 2023)**
  Summaries of real-world AE reporting and surveillance outcomes for COVID vaccines.
  Included a range of adult and pediatric populations, applying broad surveillance to detect and characterize trends in AE reporting and signal strength.

- **Obstetric Complications and Birth Outcomes After Antenatal Coronavirus Disease 2019 (COVID-19) Vaccination (Vesco et al., 2022)**
  Data-driven analysis of AEs following COVID vaccination using surveillance systems.
  Included a range of adult and pediatric populations, applying broad surveillance to detect and characterize trends in AE reporting and signal strength.

- **Post-Authorization Safety Surveillance of Ad.26.COV2.S Vaccine: Reports to the Vaccine Adverse Event Reporting System and V-safe, February 2021–February 2022 (Woo et al., 2023)**
  Summaries of real-world AE reporting and surveillance outcomes for COVID-19 vaccines.
  Included a range of adult and pediatric populations, applying broad surveillance to detect and characterize trends in AE reporting and signal strength.

- **Post-Authorization Surveillance of Adverse Events Following COVID-19 Vaccines in Pregnant Persons in the Vaccine Adverse Event Reporting System (VAERS), December 2020–October 2021 (Moro et al., 2022a)**
  Summaries of real-world AE reporting and surveillance outcomes for COVID vaccines.
  Included a range of adult and pediatric populations, applying broad surveillance to detect and characterize trends in AE reporting and signal strength.

- **Postmenopausal Bleeding After Coronavirus Disease 2019 (COVID-19) Vaccination: Vaccine Adverse Event Reporting System (Strid et al., 2022)**
  Data-driven analysis of AEs following COVID vaccination using surveillance systems.
  Included a range of adult and pediatric populations, applying broad surveillance to detect and characterize trends in AE reporting and signal strength.

APPENDIX E
213

- **Preliminary Findings of mRNA COVID-19 Vaccine Safety in Pregnant Persons (Shimabukuro et al., 2021b)**
  Data-driven analysis of AEs following COVID vaccination using surveillance systems.
  Included a range of adult and pediatric populations, applying broad surveillance to detect and characterize trends in AE reporting and signal strength.

- **Reactogenicity Following Receipt of mRNA-Based COVID-19 Vaccines (Chapin-Bardales et al., 2021a)**
  Data-driven analysis of AEs following COVID vaccination using surveillance systems.
  Included a range of adult and pediatric populations, applying broad surveillance to detect and characterize trends in AE reporting and signal strength.

- **Reactogenicity Within 2 Weeks After mRNA COVID-19 Vaccines: Findings from the CDC V-safe Surveillance System (Chapin-Bardales et al., 2021b)**
  Data-driven analysis of AEs following COVID vaccination using surveillance systems.
  Included a range of adult and pediatric populations, applying broad surveillance to detect and characterize trends in AE reporting and signal strength.

- **Reporting Rates for VAERS Death Reports Following COVID-19 Vaccination, December 14, 2020–November 17, 2021 (Day et al., 2023)**
  Data-driven analysis of AEs following COVID vaccination using surveillance systems.
  Included a range of adult and pediatric populations, applying broad surveillance to detect and characterize trends in AE reporting and signal strength.

- **Reports of Anaphylaxis After Receipt of mRNA COVID-19 Vaccines in the U.S.—December 14, 2020–January 18, 2021 (Shimabukuro et al., 2021a)**
  Data-driven analysis of AEs following COVID vaccination using surveillance systems.
  Included a range of adult and pediatric populations, applying broad surveillance to detect and characterize trends in AE reporting and signal strength.

- **Reports of Guillain-Barré Syndrome After COVID-19 Vaccination in the United States (Abara et al., 2023)**
  Data-driven analysis of AEs following COVID vaccination using surveillance systems.
  Included a range of adult and pediatric populations, applying broad surveillance to detect and characterize trends in AE reporting and signal strength.

- **Safety Monitoring of an Additional Dose of COVID-19 Vaccine—United States, August 12–September 19, 2021 (Hause et al., 2021d)**
  Summaries of real-world AE reporting and surveillance outcomes for COVID vaccines.
  Included a range of adult and pediatric populations, applying broad surveillance to detect and characterize trends in AE reporting and signal strength.

- **Safety Monitoring of Bivalent COVID-19 mRNA Vaccine Booster Doses Among Persons Aged ≥12 Years—United States, August 31–October 23, 2022 (Hause et al., 2022b)**
  Summaries of real-world AE reporting and surveillance outcomes for COVID vaccines.
  Included a range of adult and pediatric populations, applying broad surveillance to detect and characterize trends in AE reporting and signal strength.

- **Safety Monitoring of Bivalent mRNA COVID-19 Vaccine Among Pregnant Persons in the Vaccine Adverse Event Reporting System—United States, September 1, 2022–March 31, 2023 (Moro et al., 2024a)**
  Summaries of real-world AE reporting and surveillance outcomes for COVID vaccines.
  Included a range of adult and pediatric populations, applying broad surveillance to detect and characterize trends in AE reporting and signal strength.

- **Safety Monitoring of COVID-19 mRNA Vaccine First Booster Doses Among Persons Aged ≥12 Years with Presumed Immunocompromise Status—United States, January 12, 2022–March 28, 2022 (Hause et al., 2022c)**
  Summaries of real-world AE reporting and surveillance outcomes for COVID vaccines.
  Included a range of adult and pediatric populations, applying broad surveillance to detect and characterize trends in AE reporting and signal strength.

APPENDIX E 215

- Safety Monitoring of COVID-19 mRNA Vaccine Second Booster Doses Among Adults Aged ≥50 Years—United States, March 29, 2022–July 10, 2022 (Hause et al., 2022d)

  Summaries of real-world AE reporting and surveillance outcomes for COVID vaccines.

  Included a range of adult and pediatric populations, applying broad surveillance to detect and characterize trends in AE reporting and signal strength.

- Safety Monitoring of COVID-19 Vaccine Booster Doses Among Adults—United States, September 22, 2021–February 6, 2022 (Hause et al., 2022e)

  Summaries of real-world AE reporting and surveillance outcomes for COVID vaccines.

  Included a range of adult and pediatric populations, applying broad surveillance to detect and characterize trends in AE reporting and signal strength.

- Safety Monitoring of COVID-19 Vaccine Booster Doses Among Persons Aged 12–17 Years—United States, December 9, 2021–February 20, 2022 (Hause et al., 2022f)

  Summaries of real-world AE reporting and surveillance outcomes for COVID vaccines.

  Included a range of adult and pediatric populations, applying broad surveillance to detect and characterize trends in AE reporting and signal strength.

- Safety Monitoring of Pfizer-BioNTech COVID-19 Vaccine Booster Doses Among Children Aged 5–11 Years—United States, May 17–July 31, 2022 (Hause et al., 2022g)

  Summaries of real-world AE reporting and surveillance outcomes for COVID vaccines.

  Included a range of adult and pediatric populations, applying broad surveillance to detect and characterize trends in AE reporting and signal strength.

- Safety Monitoring of the Janssen (Johnson & Johnson) COVID-19 Vaccine—United States, March–April 2021 (Shay et al., 2021)

  Summaries of real-world AE reporting and surveillance outcomes for COVID vaccines.

  Included a range of adult and pediatric populations, applying broad surveillance to detect and characterize trends in AE reporting and signal strength.

- **Safety of Co-Administration of mRNA COVID-19 and Seasonal Inactivated Influenza Vaccines in the Vaccine Adverse Event Reporting System (VAERS) During July 1, 2021–June 30, 2022 (Moro et al., 2023a)**
  Data-driven analysis of AEs following COVID vaccination using surveillance systems.
  Included a range of adult and pediatric populations, applying broad surveillance to detect and characterize trends in AE reporting and signal strength.

- **Safety of mRNA Vaccines Administered During the Initial 6 Months of the U.S. COVID-19 Vaccination Programme: An Observational Study of Reports to the Vaccine Adverse Event Reporting System and V-safe (Rosenblum et al., 2022)**
  Data-driven analysis of AEs following COVID vaccination using surveillance systems.
  Included a range of adult and pediatric populations, applying broad surveillance to detect and characterize trends in AE reporting and signal strength.

- **Safety of Simultaneous Vaccination With COVID-19 Vaccines in the Vaccine Safety Datalink (Tat'Yana et al., 2023b)**
  Data-driven analysis of AEs following COVID vaccination using surveillance systems.
  Included a range of adult and pediatric populations, applying broad surveillance to detect and characterize trends in AE reporting and signal strength.

- **Surveillance for Adverse Events After COVID-19 mRNA Vaccination (Klein et al., 2021)**
  Data-driven analysis AEs following COVID vaccination using surveillance systems.
  Included a range of adult and pediatric populations, applying broad surveillance to detect and characterize trends in AE reporting and signal strength.

- **Tinnitus After COVID-19 Vaccination: Findings from the Vaccine Adverse Event Reporting System and the Vaccine Safety Datalink (Yih et al., 2024)**
  Data-driven analysis AEs following COVID vaccination using surveillance systems.
  Included a range of adult and pediatric populations, applying broad surveillance to detect and characterize trends in AE reporting and signal strength.

- **U.S. Case Reports of Cerebral Venous Sinus Thrombosis With Thrombocytopenia After Ad26.COV2.S Vaccination, March 2 to April 21, 2021 (See et al., 2021)**
  Data-driven analysis of AEs following COVID vaccination using surveillance systems.
  Included a range of adult and pediatric populations, applying broad surveillance to detect and characterize trends in AE reporting and signal strength.

ALLERGIC REACTIONS AND ANAPHYLAXIS

- **Allergic Reactions Including Anaphylaxis After Receipt of the First Dose of Moderna COVID-19 Vaccine—United States, December 21, 2020–January 10, 2021 (Shimabukuro, 2021)**
  Data-driven analysis AEs following COVID vaccination using surveillance systems.
  Focused on individuals who experienced immediate hypersensitivity reactions postvaccination, with attention to those previously sensitized to PEG-containing compounds.

- **Allergic Reactions Including Anaphylaxis After Receipt of the First Dose of Pfizer-BioNTech COVID-19 Vaccine—United States, December 14–23, 2020 (CDC, 2021)**
  Data-driven analysis of AEs following COVID vaccination using surveillance systems.
  Focused on individuals who experienced immediate hypersensitivity reactions postvaccination, with attention to those previously sensitized to PEG-containing compounds.

- **Allergic Reactions Including Anaphylaxis After Receipt of the First Dose of Pfizer-BioNTech COVID-19 Vaccine (Shimabukuro and Nair, 2021)**
  Data-driven analysis of AEs following COVID vaccination using surveillance systems.
  Focused on individuals who experienced immediate hypersensitivity reactions postvaccination, with attention to those previously sensitized to PEG-containing compounds.

- **Evaluation of Association of Anti-PEG Antibodies With Anaphylaxis After mRNA COVID-19 Vaccination (Zhou et al., 2023)**
  Evaluated potential relationship between anti-PEG antibodies and vaccine-related allergic reactions.

Focused on individuals who experienced immediate hypersensitivity reactions postvaccination, with attention to those previously sensitized to PEG-containing compounds.

BOOSTER AND BIVALENT DOSE SAFETY

- **COVID-19 Booster Vaccination in Early Pregnancy and Surveillance for Spontaneous Abortion (Kharbanda et al., 2023)**

  Evaluated safety of booster or bivalent doses in specific populations using VAERS or VSD data.

  Used VAERS and VSD to assess AEs in recipients of booster and bivalent doses, including older adults and high-risk groups.

- **Reactogenicity of Simultaneous COVID-19 mRNA Booster and Influenza Vaccination in the U.S. (Hause et al., 2022h)**

  Evaluates safety of booster or bivalent doses in specific populations using VAERS or VSD data.

  Used VAERS and VSD to assess AEs in recipients of booster and bivalent doses, including older adults and high-risk groups.

- **Safety of Booster Doses of Coronavirus Disease 2019 (COVID-19) Vaccine in Pregnancy in the Vaccine Adverse Event Reporting System (Moro et al., 2022b)**

  Evaluated safety of booster or bivalent doses in specific populations using VAERS or VSD data.

  Used VAERS and VSD to assess AEs in recipients of booster and bivalent doses, including older adults and high-risk groups.

- **Safety of Simultaneous Administration of Bivalent mRNA COVID-19 and Influenza Vaccines in the Vaccine Adverse Event Reporting System (VAERS) (Moro et al., 2024b)**

  Evaluated safety of booster or bivalent doses in specific populations using VAERS or VSD data.

  Used VAERS and VSD to assess AEs in recipients of booster and bivalent doses, including older adults and high-risk groups.

- **Safety Signal Identification for COVID-19 Bivalent Booster Vaccination Using Tree-Based Scan Statistics in the Vaccine Safety Datalink (Yih et al., 2023c)**

  Evaluates safety of booster or bivalent doses in specific populations using VAERS or VSD data.

  Used VAERS and VSD to assess AEs in recipients of booster and bivalent doses, including older adults and high-risk groups.

- Tree-Based Data Mining for Safety Assessment of First COVID-19 Booster Doses in the Vaccine Safety Datalink (Yih et al., 2023b)
  Evaluates safety of booster or bivalent doses in specific populations using VAERS or VSD data.
  Used VAERS and VSD to assess AEs in recipients of booster and bivalent doses, including older adults and high-risk groups.
  Pediatric and Adolescent Safety

- COVID-19 mRNA Vaccine Safety Among Children Aged 6 Months–5 Years—United States, June 18, 2022–August 21, 2022 (Hause et al., 2022a)
  Assessed COVID vaccine safety in pediatric or adolescent populations using active surveillance or EHR review.
  Monitored safety among children aged 5–17 years using VSD, V-safe, and VAERS, often evaluating reactogenicity and medically attended events

- COVID-19 Vaccine Safety in Adolescents Aged 12–17 Years—United States, December 14, 2020–July 16, 2021 (Hause et al., 2021b)
  Assessed COVID vaccine safety in pediatric or adolescent populations using active surveillance or EHR review.
  Monitored safety among children aged 5–17 years using VSD, V-safe, and VAERS, often evaluating reactogenicity and medically attended events.

- COVID-19 Vaccine Safety in Children Aged 5–11 Years—United States, November 3–December 19, 2021 (Hause et al., 2021c)
  Assessed COVID vaccine safety in pediatric or adolescent populations using active surveillance or EHR review.
  Monitored safety among children aged 5–17 years using VSD, V-safe, and VAERS, often evaluating reactogenicity and medically attended events.

- Reactions Following Pfizer-BioNTech COVID-19 mRNA Vaccination and Related Health Care Encounters Among 7,077 Children Aged 5–11 Years Within an Integrated Health Care System (Malden et al., 2023)
  Assessed COVID vaccine safety in pediatric or adolescent populations using active surveillance or EHR review.
  Monitored safety among children aged 5–17 years using VSD, V-safe, and VAERS, often evaluating reactogenicity and medically attended events.

- Reported Cases of Multisystem Inflammatory Syndrome in Children Aged 12–20 Years in the USA Who Received a COVID-19 Vaccine, December, 2020, Through August, 2021: A Surveillance Investigation (Yousaf et al., 2022)

Assessed COVID vaccine safety in pediatric or adolescent populations using active surveillance or EHR review.

Monitored safety among children aged 5–17 years using VSD, V-safe, and VAERS, often evaluating reactogenicity and medically attended events.

- **Safety of COVID-19 mRNA Vaccination Among Young Children in the Vaccine Safety Datalink (Goddard et al., 2023)**

  Assessed COVID vaccine safety in pediatric or adolescent populations using active surveillance or EHR review.

  Monitored safety among children aged 5–17 years using VSD, V-safe, and VAERS, often evaluating reactogenicity and medically attended events.

- **Safety of COVID-19 Vaccination in United States Children Ages 5 to 11 Years (Hause et al., 2022i)**

  Assessed COVID vaccine safety in pediatric or adolescent populations using active surveillance or EHR review.

  Monitored safety among children aged 5–17 years using VSD, V-safe, and VAERS, often evaluating reactogenicity and medically attended events.

- **Surveillance for Multisystem Inflammatory Syndrome in U.S. Children Aged 5–11 Years Who Received Pfizer-BioNTech COVID-19 Vaccine, November 2021 through March 2022 (Cortese et al., 2023)**

  Assessed COVID vaccine safety in pediatric or adolescent populations using active surveillance or EHR review.

  Monitored safety among children aged 5–17 years using VSD, V-safe, and VAERS, often evaluating reactogenicity and medically attended events.

Pregnancy Outcomes

- **COVID-19 Vaccine Safety Surveillance in Early Pregnancy in the United States: Design Factors Affecting the Association Between Vaccine and Spontaneous Abortion (Vazquez-Benitez et al., 2023)**

  Presented data-driven analysis of vaccine safety outcomes during pregnancy using registry or linked data.

  Examined pregnant individuals enrolled in V-safe or VSD, with outcomes including spontaneous abortion, stillbirth, and major birth defects.

- **Evaluation of Acute Adverse Events After COVID-19 Vaccination During Pregnancy (DeSilva et al., 2022)**

  Presented data-driven analysis of vaccine safety outcomes during pregnancy using registry or linked data.

  Examined pregnant individuals enrolled in V-safe or VSD, with outcomes including spontaneous abortion, stillbirth, and major birth defects.

- **Receipt of COVID-19 Vaccine During Pregnancy and Preterm or Small-for-Gestational-Age at Birth—Eight Integrated Health Care Organizations, United States, December 15, 2020–July 22, 2021 (Lipkind et al., 2022)**
  Presented data-driven analysis of vaccine safety outcomes during pregnancy using registry or linked data.
  Examined pregnant individuals enrolled in V-safe or VSD, with outcomes including spontaneous abortion, stillbirth, and major birth defects.

- **Spontaneous Abortion Following COVID-19 Vaccination During Pregnancy (Kharbanda et al., 2021a)**
  Presented data-driven analysis of vaccine safety outcomes during pregnancy using registry or linked data.
  Examined pregnant individuals enrolled in V-safe or VSD, with outcomes including spontaneous abortion, stillbirth, and major birth defects.

MYOCARDITIS RISK EVALUATION

- **Incidence of Myocarditis/Pericarditis Following mRNA COVID-19 Vaccination Among Children and Younger Adults in the United States (Goddard et al., 2022a)**
  Analyzed risk or incidence of myocarditis following mRNA COVID vaccination using postauthorization safety data.
  Focused primarily on adolescents and young adults, particularly male recipients, and evaluated risk after the second dose of mRNA vaccines using VAERS and VSD data.

- **Myocarditis Cases Reported After mRNA-Based COVID-19 Vaccination in the U.S. from December 2020 to August 2021 (Oster et al., 2022)**
  Analyzed risk or incidence of myocarditis following mRNA COVID vaccination using postauthorization safety data.
  Focused primarily on adolescents and young adults, particularly male recipients, and evaluated risk after the second dose of mRNA vaccines using VAERS and VSD data.

- **Myocarditis or Pericarditis Following mRNA COVID-19 Vaccination (Weintraub et al., 2022)**
  Analyzed risk or incidence of myocarditis following mRNA COVID vaccination using postauthorization safety data.
  Focused primarily on adolescents and young adults, particularly male recipients, and evaluated risk after the second dose of mRNA vaccines using VAERS and VSD data.

- **Outcomes at Least 90 Days Since Onset of Myocarditis After mRNA COVID-19 Vaccination in Adolescents and Young Adults in the USA: A Follow-Up Surveillance Study (Kracalik et al., 2022)**
  Analyzed risk or incidence of myocarditis following mRNA COVID vaccination using postauthorization safety data.
  Focused primarily on adolescents and young adults, particularly male recipients, and evaluated risk after the second dose of mRNA vaccines using VAERS and VSD data.

- **Risk of Myocarditis and Pericarditis Following BNT162b2 and mRNA-1273 COVID-19 Vaccination (Goddard et al., 2022b)**
  Analyzed risk or incidence of myocarditis following mRNA COVID vaccination using postauthorization safety data.
  Focused primarily on adolescents and young adults, particularly male recipients, and evaluated risk after the second dose of mRNA vaccines using VAERS and VSD data.

MULTISYSTEM INFLAMMATORY SYNDROME (MIS-C)

- **Multiple MIS-C Readmissions and Giant Coronary Aneurysm After COVID-19 Illness and Vaccination: A Case Report (Haq et al., 2023)**
  Surveillance and outcome characterization for MIS-C cases post-COVID or postvaccination.
  Evaluated incidence and severity of MIS-C in vaccinated versus unvaccinated children using linked hospital and vaccine records.

- **Multisystem Inflammatory Syndrome in Adults After Severe Acute Respiratory Syndrome Coronavirus 2 (SARS-CoV-2) Infection and Coronavirus Disease 2019 (COVID-19) Vaccination (Belay et al., 2022)**
  Surveillance and outcome characterization for MIS-C cases post-COVID or postvaccination.
  Evaluated incidence and severity of MIS-C in vaccinated versus unvaccinated children using linked hospital and vaccine records.

CATALOG OF DESCRIPTIVE LITERATURE FROM CDC VACCINE SAFETY MONITORING

During the COVID PHE, the ISO and its partners rapidly published a range of descriptive studies that laid the foundation for subsequent safety evaluations. These papers primarily focused on characterizing vaccine uptake, describing the function and reach of monitoring systems, and establishing the epidemiological context needed for safety signal interpretation. This body of literature did not always test hypotheses or conduct

APPENDIX E   223

comparative risk analyses but was critical in documenting population patterns, system design, and baseline expectations—especially in the early and uncertain phases of vaccine rollout.

Pregnancy Surveillance and Uptake Monitoring

Papers in this group focused on vaccine coverage, safety system implementation, and registry development for pregnant individuals—an initially excluded population in clinical trials. They leveraged VSD, VAERS, and V-safe (including the pregnancy registry) to capture postmarketing data.

- **COVID-19 Vaccination Coverage Among Pregnant Women During Pregnancy (Razzaghi et al., 2021)**
Described early vaccine uptake among pregnant individuals across VSD sites, identifying demographic disparities.
- **Monitoring the Safety of COVID-19 Vaccines in Pregnancy in the U.S. (Moro et al., 2021)**
Synthesized preliminary safety data from VAERS, VSD, and the V-safe Pregnancy Registry. No unexpected signals were noted.
- **Receipt of COVID-19 Booster Dose Among Fully Vaccinated Pregnant Individuals (Razzaghi et al., 2022)**
Provided demographic breakdowns of booster uptake in pregnant individuals, informing equity and outreach efforts.
- **CDC COVID-19 Vaccine Pregnancy Registry (Madni et al., 2024)**
Detailed design, enrollment methods, and response rates. Demonstrated feasibility of rapid registry creation during a PHE.

Equity, Demographics, and Population Coverage

These studies examined vaccine uptake and data quality across different sociodemographic groups, often using VSD infrastructure. Their value lies in identifying coverage disparities and highlighting data limitations that could bias safety signal interpretation.

- **COVID-19 Vaccination Coverage Among Insured Persons Aged ≥16 Years by Race/Ethnicity (Pingali et al., 2021)**
Tracked uptake disparities and identified subgroups with lower vaccine coverage, shaping later equity-focused communications.
- **Reporting of Race and Ethnicity in the Vaccine Safety Datalink, 2011–2022 (Kurlandsky et al., 2022)**
Assessed the completeness and trends in race/ethnicity data, critical for interpreting subgroup safety signals.

- **Association Between Vaccine Exemption Policy Change in California and Adverse Event Reporting (Hause et al., 2020)**
Provided contextual insight into how policy changes affect reporting behaviors, potentially influencing VAERS data interpretation.

Signal Detection and AE Characterization

These papers described methods and results related to identifying or contextualizing AEs of interest. While many were foundational rather than comparative, they helped build the landscape for signal evaluation.

- **Surveillance for Adverse Events After COVID-19 mRNA Vaccination (Klein et al., 2021)**
Offered early signal tracking data; documented myocarditis as a safety concern in younger males.
- **Myopericarditis After Vaccination (VAERS, 1990–2018) (Su et al., 2021)**
Placed myocarditis reports in historical context and informed comparisons to mRNA vaccine-associated rates.
- **Use of mRNA COVID-19 Vaccine After Reports of Myocarditis (ACIP Update) (Gargano et al., 2021)**
Informed risk–benefit decisions by ACIP in response to myocarditis data.
- **Tree-Based Data Mining for First Booster Doses (Yih et al., 2023b)**
Employed high-throughput signal detection methods in VSD to scan for unexpected AEs postbooster.
- **Safety Signal Identification for Bivalent Booster Vaccination (Yih et al., 2023c)**
Used tree scan methods to monitor safety in bivalent booster recipients; no new signals were observed.
- **Simultaneous Administration of Bivalent Booster and Influenza Vaccines (Tat'Yana et al., 2023a)**
Evaluated safety of coadministration; important for fall campaign planning.
- **Updated Recommendations for Janssen Vaccine After TTS Reports (MacNeil et al., 2021)**
Summarized evidence on thrombosis with thrombocytopenia syndrome and associated policy response.
- **Causality Assessment of Adverse Events Reported to VAERS (Loughlin et al., 2012)**
Described approaches for interpreting spontaneous reports, laying groundwork for postmarketing review methodology.

- **Algorithm to Assess Causality After Individual Adverse Events Following Immunizations (Halsey et al., 2012)**
  Outlined systematic methods for determining vaccine-attributable events using structured criteria.

System Infrastructure and Data Tools

These publications described the design, function, and capabilities of CDC's vaccine safety surveillance systems, such as VAERS, VSD, V-safe, and CISA. While not evaluative of safety itself, they were essential for understanding system architecture and integration during the COVID response.

- **Overview of U.S. COVID-19 Vaccine Safety Surveillance Systems (Gee et al., 2024)**
  Summarized the scope, coordination, and role of each system in the national safety monitoring strategy.
- **The V-safe After Vaccination Health Checker (Moro et al., 2023b)**
  Provided early operational results from V-safe, including enrollment and symptom reporting patterns.
- **Impact of the COVID-19 Pandemic on Health Care Utilization in the Vaccine Safety Datalink (Qian et al., 2024)**
  Described changes in data quality and patterns that could affect VSD-based analyses.
- **Dashboard Development for Real-Time Visualization of VSD Safety Data (Tat'Yana et al., 2022)**
  Highlighted innovations in visualizing vaccine safety data for internal and external stakeholders.
- **Overview of the Clinical Consult Case Review Network (CISA) (Williams et al., 2011)**
  Provided historical and operational background on CISA's role in managing complex clinical safety consultations.
- **A Decade of Data: Adolescent Vaccination in VSD (Irving et al., 2022)**
  While pre-COVID, this paper demonstrated VSD's capacity for long-term safety monitoring in a specific population.
- **Reporting Sensitivity of VAERS for Anaphylaxis and Guillain-Barré Syndrome (Miller et al., 2020)**
  Quantified the underreporting in VAERS for two serious AEs, helping contextualize COVID signal detection sensitivity.
- **Understanding the Role of Human Variation in Vaccine Adverse Events (CISA) (LaRussa et al., 2011)**
  Offered insights into host-specific factors that could contribute to AE risk—relevant to interpreting heterogeneity in COVID AE patterns.

Methodological Tools and Epidemiologic Context

These studies supported vaccine safety interpretation by developing background incidence rates, refining analytic techniques, and highlighting future methodological needs.

- **Novel Vaccine Safety Issues and Areas for Further Research (Salmon et al., 2021)**
Outlined thematic gaps in safety knowledge and future directions, including long-term and rare event monitoring.
- **Expected Rates of Select Adverse Events Following Immunization (Abara et al., 2022)**
Provided critical baseline rates to assess observed-to-expected event ratios—central for VAERS signal evaluation.
- **Developing Algorithms for Birth Defect Detection Using EHR Data (Kharbanda et al., 2021b)**
Demonstrated a scalable approach to detecting structural birth defects—a key outcome of interest for pregnancy safety monitoring.
- **COVID-19 Vaccine Safety Inquiries to the CDC ISO (Miller et al., 2023)**
Catalogued inquiries and communication trends received by ISO, helping shape transparency and messaging strategies.

REFERENCES

Abara, W. E., J. Gee, M. Delorey, Y. Tun, Y. Mu, D. K. Shay, and T. Shimabukuro. 2022. Expected rates of select adverse events after immunization for coronavirus disease 2019 vaccine safety monitoring. *Journal of Infectious Diseases* 225(9):1569–1574. https://doi.org/10.1093/infdis/jiab628.

Abara, W. E., J. Gee, P. Marquez, J. Woo, T. R. Myers, A. DeSantis, J. A. Baumblatt, E. J. Woo, D. Thompson, and N. Nair. 2023. Reports of Guillain-Barré syndrome after COVID-19 vaccination in the United States. *JAMA Network Open* 6(2):e2253845. https://doi.org/10.1001/jamanetworkopen.2022.53845.

Belay, E. D., S. Godfred Cato, A. K. Rao, J. Abrams, W. Wyatt Wilson, S. Lim, C. Newton-Cheh, M. Melgar, J. DeCuir, and B. Webb. 2022. Multisystem inflammatory syndrome in adults after severe acute respiratory syndrome coronavirus 2 (SARS-CoV-2) infection and coronavirus disease 2019 (COVID-19) vaccination. *Clinical Infectious Diseases* 75(1):e741–e748. https://doi.org/10.1093/cid/ciab936.

CDC (Centers for Disease Control and Prevention). 2021. Allergic reactions including anaphylaxis after receipt of the first dose of Pfizer-BioNTech COVID-19 vaccine—United States, December 14–23, 2020.

Chapin-Bardales, J., J. Gee, and T. Myers. 2021a. Reactogenicity following receipt of mRNA-based COVID-19 vaccines. *JAMA* 325(21):2201–2202. https://doi.org/10.1001/jama.2021.5374.

Chapin-Bardales, J., T. Myers, J. Gee, D. K. Shay, P. Marquez, J. Baggs, B. Zhang, C. Licata, and T. T. Shimabukuro. 2021b. Reactogenicity within 2 weeks after mRNA COVID-19 vaccines: Findings from the CDC V-safe Surveillance System. *Vaccine* 39(48):7066. https://doi.org/10.1016/j.vaccine.2021.10.019.

Cortese, M. M., A. W. Taylor, L. J. Akinbami, A. Thames-Allen, A. R. Yousaf, A. P. Campbell, S. A. Maloney, T. A. Harrington, E. G. Anyalechi, and D. Munshi. 2023. Surveillance for multisystem inflammatory syndrome in U.S. children aged 5–11 years who received Pfizer-BioNTech COVID-19 vaccine, November 2021 through March 2022. *Journal of Infectious Diseases* 228(2):143–148. https://doi.org/10.1093/infdis/jiad051.
Day, B., D. Menschik, D. Thompson, C. Jankosky, J. Su, P. Moro, C. Zinderman, K. Welsh, R. B. Dimova, and N. Nair. 2023. Reporting rates for VAERS death reports following COVID-19 vaccination, December 14, 2020–November 17, 2021. *Pharmacoepidemiology and Drug Safety* 32(7):763–772. https://doi.org/10.1002/pds.5605.
DeSilva, M., J. Haapala, G. Vazquez-Benitez, K. K. Vesco, M. F. Daley, D. Getahun, O. Zerbo, A. Naleway, J. C. Nelson, and J. T. Williams. 2022. Evaluation of acute adverse events after COVID-19 vaccination during pregnancy. *New England Journal of Medicine* 387(2):187–189. https://doi.org/10.1056/NEJMc2205276.
Gargano, J. W., M. Wallace, S. C. Hadler, G. Langley, J. R. Su, M. E. Oster, K. R. Broder, J. Gee, E. Weintraub, T. Shimabukuro, H. M. Scobie, D. Moulia, L. E. Markowitz, M. Wharton, V. V. McNally, J. R. Romero, H. K. Talbot, G. M. Lee, M. F. Daley, and S. E. Oliver. 2021. Use of mRNA COVID-19 vaccine after reports of myocarditis among vaccine recipients: Update from the Advisory Committee on Immunization Practices—United States, June 2021. *MMWR* 70(27):977–982. https://doi.org/10.15585/mmwr.mm7027e2.
Gee, J., P. Marquez, J. R. Su, G. M. Calvert, R. Liu, T. R. Myers, N. Nair, S. Martin, T. Clark, L. E. Markowitz, N. Lindsey, B. Zhang, C. Licata, A. Jazwa, M. Sotir, and T. Shimabukuro 2021. First month of COVID-19 vaccine safety monitoring—United States, December 14, 2020–January 13, 2021. *MMWR*. https://doi.org/7010.15585/mmwr.mm7008e3.
Gee, J., T. T. Shimabukuro, J. R. Su, D. Shay, M. Ryan, S. V. Basavaraju, K. R. Broder, M. Clark, C. B. Creech, and F. Cunningham. 2024. Overview of U.S. COVID-19 vaccine safety surveillance systems. *Vaccine* 42:125748.
Goddard, K., K. E. Hanson, N. Lewis, E. Weintraub, B. Fireman, and N. P. Klein. 2022a. Incidence of myocarditis/pericarditis following mRNA COVID-19 vaccination among children and younger adults in the United States. *Annals of Internal Medicine* 175(11):1169–1771.
Goddard, K., N. Lewis, B. Fireman, E. Weintraub, T. Shimabukuro, O. Zerbo, T. G. Boyce, M. E. Oster, K. E. Hanson, and J. G. Donahue. 2022b. Risk of myocarditis and pericarditis following BNT162B2 and mRNA-1273 COVID-19 vaccination. *Vaccine* 40(35):5153–5159. https://doi.org/10.1016/j.vaccine.2022.07.007.
Goddard, K., J. G. Donahue, N. Lewis, K. E. Hanson, E. S. Weintraub, B. Fireman, and N. P. Klein. 2023. Safety of COVID-19 mRNA vaccination among young children in the Vaccine Safety Datalink. *Pediatrics* 152(1). https://doi.org/10.1542/peds.2023-061894.
Halsey, N. A., K. M. Edwards, C. L. Dekker, N. P. Klein, R. Baxter, P. Larussa, C. Marchant, B. Slade, C. Vellozzi, and the Causality Working Group of the Clinical Immunization Safety Assessment Network. 2012. Algorithm to assess causality after individual adverse events following immunizations. *Vaccine* 30(39):5791–5798. https://doi.org/10.1016/j.vaccine.2012.04.005.
Hanson, K. E., K. Goddard, N. Lewis, B. Fireman, T. R. Myers, N. Bakshi, E. Weintraub, J. G. Donahue, J. C. Nelson, and S. Xu. 2021. Guillain-Barré syndrome after COVID-19 vaccination in the Vaccine Safety Datalink. https://doi.org/10.1001/jamanetworkopen.2022.8879.
Hanson, K. E., K. Goddard, N. Lewis, B. Fireman, T. R. Myers, N. Bakshi, E. Weintraub, J. G. Donahue, J. C. Nelson, and S. Xu. 2022. Incidence of Guillain-Barré syndrome after COVID-19 vaccination in the Vaccine Safety Datalink. *JAMA Network Open* 5(4):e228879. https://doi.org/10.1001/jamanetworkopen.2022.8879.
Haq, K., E. G. Anyalechi, E. P. Schlaudecker, R. McKay, S. Kamidani, C. K. Manos, and M. E. Oster. 2023. Multiple MIS-C readmissions and giant coronary aneurysm after COVID-19 illness and vaccination: A case report. *Pediatric Infectious Disease Journal* 42(3):e64–e69. https://doi.org/10.1097/INF.0000000000003801.

Hause, A. M., E. M. Hesse, C. Ng, P. Marquez, M. M. McNeil, and S. B. Omer. 2020. Association between vaccine exemption policy change in California and adverse event reporting. *Pediatric Infectious Disease Journal* 39(5):369–373. https://doi.org/10.1097/INF.0000000000002585.

Hause, A. M. 2021a. Anxiety-related adverse event clusters after Janssen COVID-19 vaccination—five U.S. mass vaccination sites, April 2021. *MMWR* 70. https://doi.org/10.15585/mmwr.mm7018e3.

Hause, A. M., J. Gee, J. Baggs, W. E. Abara, P. Marquez, D. Thompson, J. R. Su, C. Licata, H. G. Rosenblum, T. R. Myers, T. Shimabukuro, and D. Shay. 2021b. COVID-19 vaccine safety in adolescents aged 12–17 years—United States, December 14, 2020–July 16, 2021. *MMWR* 70.

Hause, A. M., J. Baggs, P. Marquez, T. R. Myers, J. Gee, J. R. Su, B. Zhang, D. Thompson, T. Shimabukuro, and D. Shay. 2021c. COVID-19 vaccine safety in children aged 5–11 years—United States, November 3–December 19, 2021. *MMWR* 70.

Hause, A. M., J. Baggs, J. Gee, P. Marquez, T.R. Myers, T. Shimabukuro, D. K. Shay. 2021d. Safety monitoring of an additional dose of COVID-19 vaccine—United States, August 12–September 19, 2021. *MMWR* 70. https://doi.org/10.15585/mmwr.mm7039e4.

Hause, A. M., P. Marquez, B. Zhang, T. R. Myers, J. Gee, J. R. Su, C. Parker, D. Thompson, S. S. Panchanathan, T. Shimabukuro, and D. Shay. 2022a. COVID-19 mRNA vaccine safety among children aged 6 months–5 years—United States, June 18, 2022–August 21, 2022. *MMWR* 71. https://doi.org/10.15585/mmwr.mm7135a3.

Hause, A. M., P. Marquez, B. Zhang, T. R. Myers, J. Gee, J. R. Su, P. G. Blanc, A. Thomas, D. Thompson, T. Shimabukuro, and D. Shay. 2022b. Safety monitoring of bivalent COVID-19 mRNA vaccine booster doses among persons aged ≥12 years—United States, August 31–October 23, 2022. *MMWR* 71. https://doi.org/10.15585/mmwr.mm7144a3.

Hause, A. M., J. Baggs, P. Marquez, W. E. Abara, J. G. Baumblatt, D. Thompson, J. R. Su, T. R. Myers, J. Gee, T. Shimabukuro, and D. Shay. 2022c. Safety monitoring of COVID-19 mRNA vaccine first booster doses among persons aged ≥12 years with presumed immunocompromise status—United States, January 12, 2022–March 28, 2022. *MMWR* 71. https://doi.org/10.15585/mmwr.mm7128a3.

Hause, A. M., J. Baggs, P. Marquez, W. E. Abara, J. G. Baumblatt, P. G. Blanc, J. R. Su, B. Hugueley, C. Parker, T. R. Myers, J. Gee, T. Shimabukuro, and D. Shay. 2022d. Safety monitoring of COVID-19 mRNA vaccine second booster doses among adults aged ≥50 years—United States, March 29, 2022–July 10, 2022. *MMWR* 71. https://doi.org/10.15585/mmwr.mm7130a4.

Hause, A. M., J. Baggs, P. Marquez, T. R. Myers, J. R. Su, P. G. Blanc, J. G. Baumblatt, E. J. Woo, J. Gee, T. Shimabukuro, and D. Shay. 2022e. Safety monitoring of COVID-19 vaccine booster doses among adults—United States, September 22, 2021–February 6, 2022. *MMWR* 71. https://doi.org/10.15585/mmwr.mm7107e1.

Hause, A. M., J. Baggs, P. Marquez, W. E. Abara, B. Olubajo, T. R. Myers, J. R. Su, D. Thompson, J. Gee, T. Shimabukuro, and D. Shay. 2022f. Safety monitoring of COVID-19 vaccine booster doses among persons aged 12–17 years—United States, December 9, 2021–February 20, 2022. *MMWR* 71. https://doi.org/10.15585/mmwr.mm7109e2.

Hause, A. M., J. Baggs, P. Marquez, T. R. Myers, J. R. Su, B. Hugueley, D. Thompson, J. Gee, T. Shimabukuro, and D. Shay. 2022g. Safety monitoring of Pfizer-BioNTech COVID-19 vaccine booster doses among children aged 5–11 years—United States, May 17–July 31, 2022. *MMWR* 71. https://doi.org/10.15585/mmwr.mm7133a3.

Hause, A. M., D. K. Shay, N. P. Klein, W. E. Abara, J. Baggs, M. M. Cortese, B. Fireman, J. Gee, J. M. Glanz, and K. Goddard. 2022h. Safety of COVID-19 vaccination in United States children ages 5 to 11 years. *Pediatrics* 150(2). https://doi.org/10.1542/peds.2022-057313.

Hause, A. M., B. Zhang, X. Yue, P. Marquez, T. R. Myers, C. Parker, J. Gee, J. Su, T. T. Shimabukuro, and D. K. Shay. 2022i. Reactogenicity of simultaneous COVID-19 mRNA booster and influenza vaccination in the U.S. *JAMA Network Open* 5(7):e2222241. https://doi.org/10.1001/jamanetworkopen.2022.22241.

Irving, S. A., H. C. Groom, P. Dandamudi, M. F. Daley, J. G. Donahue, J. Gee, R. Hechter, L. A. Jackson, N. P. Klein, E. Liles, T. R. Myers, and S. Stokley. 2022. A decade of data: Adolescent vaccination in the Vaccine Safety Datalink, 2007 through 2016. *Vaccine* 40(9):1246–1252. https://doi.org/10.1016/j.vaccine.2022.01.051.

Kharbanda, E. O., J. Haapala, M. DeSilva, G. Vazquez-Benitez, K. K. Vesco, A. L. Naleway, and H. S. Lipkind. 2021a. Spontaneous abortion following COVID-19 vaccination during pregnancy. *JAMA* 326(16):1629–1631. https://doi.org/10.1001/jama.2021.15494.

Kharbanda, E. O., G. Vazquez-Benitez, M. B. DeSilva, A. B. Spaulding, M. F. Daley, A. L. Naleway, S. A. Irving, N. P. Klein, H. F. Tseng, and L. A. Jackson. 2021b. Developing algorithms for identifying major structural birth defects using automated electronic health data. *Pharmacoepidemiology and Drug Safety* 30(2):266–274.

Kharbanda, E. O., J. Haapala, H. S. Lipkind, M. B. DeSilva, J. Zhu, K. K. Vesco, M. F. Daley, J. G. Donahue, D. Getahun, and S. J. Hambidge. 2023. COVID-19 booster vaccination in early pregnancy and surveillance for spontaneous abortion. *JAMA Network Open* 6(5):e2314350. https://doi.org/10.1001/jamanetworkopen.2023.14350.

Klein, N. P., N. Lewis, K. Goddard, B. Fireman, O. Zerbo, K. E. Hanson, J. G. Donahue, E. O. Kharbanda, A. Naleway, J. C. Nelson, S. Xu, W. K. Yih, J. M. Glanz, J. T. B. Williams, S. J. Hambidge, B. J. Lewin, T. T. Shimabukuro, F. DeStefano, and E. S. Weintraub. 2021. Surveillance for adverse events after COVID-19 mRNA vaccination. *JAMA* 326(14):1390–1399. https://doi.org/10.1001/jama.2021.15072.

Kracalik, I., M. E. Oster, K. R. Broder, M. M. Cortese, M. Glover, K. Shields, C. B. Creech, B. Romanson, S. Novosad, and J. Soslow. 2022. Outcomes at least 90 days since onset of myocarditis after mRNA COVID-19 vaccination in adolescents and young adults in the USA: A follow-up surveillance study. *Lancet Child & Adolescent Health* 6(11):788–798. https://doi.org/10.1016/S2352-4642(22)00244-9.

Kurlandsky, K., S. J. Hambidge, E. Weintraub, and J. T. Williams. 2022. Reporting of race and ethnicity in the Vaccine Safety Datalink, 2011–2021. Paper read at APHA 2022 Annual Meeting and Expo.

LaRussa, P. S., K. M. Edwards, C. L. Dekker, N. P. Klein, N. A. Halsey, C. Marchant, R. Baxter, R. J. Engler, J. Kissner, and B. A. Slade. 2011. Understanding the role of human variation in vaccine adverse events: The Clinical Immunization Safety Assessment network. *Pediatrics* 127(Supplement_1):S65–S73. https://doi.org/10.1542/peds.2010-1722J.

Lipkind, H. S., G. Vasquez-Benitez, M. DeSilva, K. K. Vesco, K. Ackerman-Banks, J. Zhu, T. G. Boyce, M. F. Daley, C. C. Fuller, D. Getahun, S. A. Irving, L. Jackson, J. T. B. Williams, O. Zerbo, M. M. McNeil, C. Olson, E. Weintraub, and E. O. Kharbanda. 2022. Receipt of COVID-19 vaccine during pregnancy and preterm or small-for-gestational-age at birth—eight integrated health care organizations, United States, December 15, 2020–July 22, 2021. *MMWR* 71. https://doi.org/10.15585/mmwr.mm7101e1.

Loughlin, A. M., C. D. Marchant, W. Adams, E. Barnett, R. Baxter, S. Black, C. Casey, C. Dekker, K. M. Edwards, J. Klein, N. P. Klein, P. LaRussa, R. Sparks, and K. Jakob. 2012. Causality assessment of adverse events reported to the Vaccine Adverse Event Reporting System (VAERS). *Vaccine* 30(50):7253–7259. https://doi.org/10.1016/j.vaccine.2012.09.074.

MacNeil, J. R., J. R. Su, K. R. Broder, A. Y. Guh, J. W. Gargano, M. Wallace, S. C. Hadler, H. M. Scobie, A. E. Blain, D. Moulia, M. F. Daley, V. V. McNally, J. R. Romero, H. K. Talbot, G. M. Lee, B. P. Bell, and S. E. Oliver. 2021. Updated recommendations from the Advisory Committee on Immunization Practices for use of the Janssen (Johnson & Johnson) COVID-19 vaccine after reports of thrombosis with thrombocytopenia syndrome among vaccine recipients—United States, April 2021. *MMWR* 70(17):651–656. https://doi.org/10.15585/mmwr.mm7017e4.

Madni, S. A., A. J. Sharma, L. H. Zauche, A. V. Waters, J. F. Nahabedian, 3rd, T. Johnson, C. K. Olson, and CDC COVID-19 Vaccine Pregnancy Registry Work Group. 2024. CDC COVID-19 Vaccine Pregnancy Registry: Design, data collection, response rates, and cohort description. *Vaccine* 42(7):1469–1477. https://doi.org/10.1016/j.vaccine.2023.11.061.

Malden, D. E., J. Gee, S. Glenn, Z. Li, C. Mercado, O. A. Ogun, S. Kim, B. J. Lewin, B. K. Ackerson, and A. Jazwa. 2023. Reactions following Pfizer-BioNTech COVID-19 mRNA vaccination and related healthcare encounters among 7,077 children aged 5–11 years within an integrated healthcare system. *Vaccine* 41(2):315–322. https://doi.org/10.1016/j.vaccine.2022.10.079.

Miller, E. R., M. M. McNeil, P. L. Moro, J. Duffy, and J. R. Su. 2020. The reporting sensitivity of the Vaccine Adverse Event Reporting System (VAERS) for anaphylaxis and for Guillain-Barre Syndrome. *Vaccine* 38(47):7458–7463. https://doi.org/10.1016/j.vaccine.2020.09.072.

Miller, E. R., P. L. Moro, T. T. Shimabukuro, G. Carlock, S. N. Davis, E. M. Freeborn, A. L. Roberts, J. Gee, A. W. Taylor, R. Gallego, T. Suragh, and J. R. Su. 2023. COVID-19 vaccine safety inquiries to the Centers for Disease Control and Prevention Immunization Safety Office. *Vaccine* 41(27):3960–3963. https://doi.org/10.1016/j.vaccine.2023.05.054.

Moro, P. L., L. Panagiotakopoulos, T. Oduyebo, C. K. Olson, and T. Myers. 2021. Monitoring the safety of COVID-19 vaccines in pregnancy in the U.S. *Human Vaccines & Immunotherapeutics* 17(12):4705–4713.

Moro, P. L., C. K. Olson, E. Clark, P. Marquez, P. Strid, S. Ellington, B. Zhang, A. Mba-Jonas, M. Alimchandani, and J. Cragan. 2022a. Post-authorization surveillance of adverse events following COVID-19 vaccines in pregnant persons in the Vaccine Adverse Event Reporting System (VAERS), December 2020–October 2021. *Vaccine* 40(24):3389–3394. https://doi.org/10.1016/j.vaccine.2022.04.031.

Moro, P. L., C. K. Olson, B. Zhang, P. Marquez, and P. Strid. 2022b. Safety of booster doses of coronavirus disease 2019 (COVID-19) vaccine in pregnancy in the Vaccine Adverse Event Reporting System. *Obstetrics & Gynecology* 140(3):421–427. https://doi.org/10.1097/AOG.0000000000004889.

Moro, P. L., B. Zhang, C. Ennulat, M. Harris, R. McVey, G. Woody, P. Marquez, M. M. McNeil, and J. R. Su. 2023a. Safety of co-administration of mRNA COVID-19 and seasonal inactivated influenza vaccines in the Vaccine Adverse Event Reporting System (VAERS) during July 1, 2021–June 30, 2022. *Vaccine* 41(11):1859–1863. https://doi.org/10.1016/j.vaccine.2022.12.069.

Moro, P. L., B. Zhang, C. Ennulat, M. Harris, R. McVey, G. Woody, P. Marquez, M. M. McNeil, and J. Myers, T. R., P. L. Marquez, J. M. Gee, A. M. Hause, L. Panagiotakopoulos, B. Zhang, I. McCullum, C. Licata, C. K. Olson, S. Rahman, S. B. Kennedy, M. Cardozo, C. R. Patel, L. Maxwell, J. R. Kallman, D. K. Shay, and T. T. Shimabukuro. 2023b. The V-Safe after vaccination health checker: Active vaccine safety monitoring during CDC's COVID-19 pandemic response. *Vaccine* 41(7):1310–1318. https://doi.org/10.1016/j.vaccine.2022.12.031.

Moro, P. L., G. Carlock, N. Fifadara, T. Habenicht, B. Zhang, P. Strid, and P. Marquez. 2024a. Safety monitoring of bivalent mRNA COVID-19 vaccine among pregnant persons in the Vaccine Adverse Event Reporting System–United States, September 1, 2022–March 31, 2023. *Vaccine* 42(9):2380–2384. https://doi.org/10.1016/j.vaccine.2024.02.084.

Moro, P. L., C. Ennulat, H. Brown, G. Woody, B. Zhang, P. Marquez, E. J. Woo, and J. R. Su. 2024b. Safety of simultaneous administration of bivalent mRNA COVID-19 and influenza vaccines in the Vaccine Adverse Event Reporting System (VAERS). *Drug Safety* 47(5):487–493. https://doi.org/10.1007/s40264-024-01406-8.

Oster, M. E., D. K. Shay, J. R. Su, J. Gee, C. B. Creech, K. R. Broder, K. Edwards, J. H. Soslow, J. M. Dendy, and E. Schlaudecker. 2022. Myocarditis cases reported after mRNA-based COVID-19 vaccination in the U.S. from December 2020 to August 2021. *JAMA* 327(4):331–340. https://doi.org/10.1001/jama.2021.24110.

Pingali, C., M. Meghani, H. Razzaghi, M. J. Lamias, E. Weintraub, T. A. Kenigsberg, J. Klein, N. Lewis, B. Fireman, O. Zerbo, J. Bartlett, K. Goddard, J. Donahue, K. E. Hanson, A. Naleway, E. O. Kharbanda, W. K. Yih, J. Nelson, B. J. Lewin, J. T. B. Williams, J. M. Glanz, J. A. Singleton, and S. A. Patel. 2021. COVID-19 vaccination coverage among insured persons aged ≥ 16 years, by race/ethnicity and other selected characteristics—eight integrated health care organizations, United States, December 14, 2020–May 15, 2021. *MMWR* 70(28):985–990. https://doi.org/10.15585/mmwr.mm7028a1.

Qian, L., L. S. Sy, V. Hong, S. C. Glenn, D. S. Ryan, J. C. Nelson, S. J. Hambidge, B. Crane, O. Zerbo, and M. B. DeSilva. 2024. Impact of the COVID-19 pandemic on health care utilization in the Vaccine Safety Datalink: Retrospective cohort study. *JMIR Public Health and Surveillance* 10(1):e48159. https://doi.org/10.2196/48159.

Razzaghi, H., M. Meghani, C. Pingali, B. Crane, A. Naleway, E. Weintraub, T. A. Kenigsberg, M. J. Lamias, S. A. Irving, T. L. Kauffman, K. K. Vesco, M. F. Daley, M. DeSilva, J. Donahue, D. Getahun, S. Glenn, S. J. Hambidge, L. Jackson, H. S. Lipkind, J. Nelson, O. Zerbo, T. Oduyebo, J. A. Singleton, and S. A. Patel. 2021. COVID-19 vaccination coverage among pregnant women during pregnancy—eight integrated health care organizations, United States, December 14, 2020–May 8, 2021. *MMWR* 70(24):895–899. https://doi.org/10.15585/mmwr.mm7024e2.

Razzaghi, H., M. Meghani, B. Crane, S. Ellington, A. L. Naleway, S. A. Irving, and S. A. Patel. 2022. Receipt of COVID-19 booster dose among fully vaccinated pregnant individuals aged 18 to 49 years by key demographics. *JAMA* 327(23):2351–2354.

Romanson, B., P. Moro, J. R. Su, P. Marquez, N. Nair, B. Day, A. DeSantis, and T. Shimabukuro. 2023. Notes from the field: Safety monitoring of novavax COVID-19 vaccine among persons aged ≥12 years—United States, July 13, 2022–March 13, 2023. *MMWR* 72. https://doi.org/10.15585/mmwr.mm7231a4.

Rosenblum, H. G., J. Gee, R. Liu, P. L. Marquez, B. Zhang, P. Strid, W. E. Abara, M. M. McNeil, T. R. Myers, and A. M. Hause. 2022. Safety of mRNA vaccines administered during the initial 6 months of the U.S. COVID-19 vaccination programme: An observational study of reports to the Vaccine Adverse Event Reporting System and V-safe. *Lancet Infectious Diseases* 22(6):802–8120. https://doi.org/1016/S1473-3099(22)00054-8.

Salmon, Daniel A., Paul Henry Lambert, Hanna M. Nohynek, Julianne Gee, Umesh D. Parashar, Jacqueline E. Tate, Annelies Wilder-Smith, Kenneth Y. Hatigan-Go, Peter G. Smith, Patrick Louis F. Zuber. 2021. Novel vaccine safety issues and areas that would benefit from further research. *BMJ Global Health*. https://doi.org/10.1136/bmjgh-2020-003814.

See, I., J. R. Su, A. Lale, E. J. Woo, A. Y. Guh, T. T. Shimabukuro, M. B. Streiff, A. K. Rao, A. P. Wheeler, and S. F. Beavers. 2021. U.S. case reports of cerebral venous sinus thrombosis with thrombocytopenia after AD26. CoV2. S vaccination, March 2 to April 21, 2021. *JAMA* 325(24):2448–2456. https://doi.org/10.1001/jama.2021.7517.

See, I., A. Lale, P. Marquez, M. B. Streiff, A. P. Wheeler, N. K. Tepper, E. J. Woo, K. R. Broder, K. M. Edwards, and R. Gallego. 2022. Case series of thrombosis with thrombocytopenia syndrome after COVID-19 vaccination—United States, December 2020 to August 2021. *Annals of Internal Medicine* 175(4):513–522. https://doi.org/10.7326/M21-4502.

Shay, D. K., J. Gee, J. R. Su, T. R. Myers, P. Marquez, R. Liu, B. Zhang, C. Licata, T. A. Clark, and T. Shimabukuro. 2021. Safety monitoring of the Janssen (Johnson & Johnson) COVID-19 vaccine—United States, March–April 2021. *MMWR* 70. https://doi.org/10.15585/mmwr.mm7018e2.

Shimabukuro, T. 2021. Allergic reactions including anaphylaxis after receipt of the first dose of Moderna COVID-19 vaccine—United States, December 21, 2020–January 10, 2021. *American Journal of Transplantation* 21(3):1326–1331. https://doi.org/10.1111/ajt.16517.

Shimabukuro, T., and N. Nair. 2021. Allergic reactions including anaphylaxis after receipt of the first dose of Pfizer-BioNTech COVID-19 vaccine. *JAMA* 325(8):780–781. https://doi.org/10.1001/jama.2021.0600.

Shimabukuro, T. T., M. Cole, and J. R. Su. 2021a. Reports of anaphylaxis after receipt of mRNA COVID-19 vaccines in the U.S.—December 14, 2020–January 18, 2021. *JAMA* 325(11):1101–1102. https://doi.org/10.1001/jama.2021.1967.

Shimabukuro, T. T., S. Y. Kim, T. R. Myers, P. L. Moro, T. Oduyebo, L. Panagiotakopoulos, P. L. Marquez, C. K. Olson, R. Liu, and K. T. Chang. 2021b. Preliminary findings of mRNA COVID-19 vaccine safety in pregnant persons. *New England Journal of Medicine* 384(24):2273–2282. https://doi.org/10.1056/NEJMoa2104983.

Strid, P., W. E. Abara, E. Clark, P. L. Moro, C. K. Olson, and J. Gee. 2022. Postmenopausal bleeding after coronavirus disease 2019 (COVID-19) vaccination: Vaccine Adverse Event Reporting System. *Obstetrics & Gynecology*. https://doi.org/10.109710.1097/AOG.0000000000005615.

Su, J. R., M. M. McNeil, K. J. Welsh, P. L. Marquez, C. Ng, M. Yan, and M. V. Cano. 2021. Myopericarditis after vaccination, Vaccine Adverse Event Reporting System (VAERS), 1990–2018. *Vaccine* 39(5):839–845. https://doi.org/10.1016/j.vaccine.2020.12.046.

Tat'Yana, A. K., A. M. Hause, M. M. McNeil, J. C. Nelson, J. A. Shoup, K. Goddard, Y. Lou, K. E. Hanson, S. C. Glenn, and E. S. Weintraub. 2022. Dashboard development for near real-time visualization of COVID-19 vaccine safety surveillance data in the Vaccine Safety Datalink. *Vaccine* 40(22):3064–3071.

Tat'Yana, A. K., K. Goddard, K. E. Hanson, N. Lewis, N. Klein, S. A. Irving, A. L. Naleway, B. Crane, T. L. Kauffman, and S. Xu. 2023a. Simultaneous administration of mRNA COVID-19 bivalent booster and influenza vaccines. *Vaccine* 41(39):5678–5682.

Tat'Yana, A. K., K. E. Hanson, N. P. Klein, O. Zerbo, K. Goddard, S. Xu, W. K. Yih, S. A. Irving, L. P. Hurley, and J. M. Glanz. 2023b. Safety of simultaneous vaccination with COVID-19 vaccines in the Vaccine Safety Datalink. *Vaccine* 41(32):4658–4665. https://doi.org/10.1016/j.vaccine.2023.06.042.

Tompkins, L. K., J. Baggs, T. R. Myers, J. M. Gee, P. L. Marquez, S. B. Kennedy, D. Peake, D. Dua, A. M. Hause, and P. Strid. 2022. Association between history of SARS-CoV-2 infection and severe systemic adverse events after mRNA COVID-19 vaccination among U.S. adults. *Vaccine* 40(52):7653–7659. https://doi.org/10.1016/j.vaccine.2022.10.073.

Vazquez-Benitez, G., J. L. Haapala, H. S. Lipkind, M. B. DeSilva, J. Zhu, M. F. Daley, D. Getahun, N. P. Klein, K. K. Vesco, and S. A. Irving. 2023. COVID-19 vaccine safety surveillance in early pregnancy in the United States: Design factors affecting the association between vaccine and spontaneous abortion. *American Journal of Epidemiology* 192(8):1386–1395. https://doi.org/10.1093/aje/kwad059.

Vesco, K. K., A. E. Denoble, H. S. Lipkind, E. O. Kharbanda, M. B. DeSilva, M. F. Daley, D. Getahun, O. Zerbo, A. L. Naleway, and L. Jackson. 2022. Obstetric complications and birth outcomes after antenatal coronavirus disease 2019 (COVID-19) vaccination. *Obstetrics & Gynecology*. https://doi.org/10.109710.1097/AOG.0000000000005583.

Weintraub, E. S., M. E. Oster, and N. P. Klein. 2022. Myocarditis or pericarditis following mRNA COVID-19 vaccination. *JAMA Network Open* 5(6):e2218512. https://doi.org/10.1001/jamanetworkopen.2022.18512.

Williams, S. E., N. P. Klein, N. Halsey, C. L. Dekker, R. P. Baxter, C. D. Marchant, P. S. LaRussa, R. C. Sparks, J. I. Tokars, and B. A. Pahud. 2011. Overview of the clinical consult case review of adverse events following immunization: Clinical Immunization Safety Assessment (CISA) network 2004–2009. *Vaccine* 29(40):6920–6927.

Wong, K. K., C. M. Heilig, A. Hause, T. R. Myers, C. K. Olson, J. Gee, P. Marquez, P. Strid, and D. K. Shay. 2022. Menstrual irregularities and vaginal bleeding after COVID-19 vaccination reported to V-safe active surveillance, USA in December, 2020–January, 2022: An observational cohort study. *Lancet Digital Health* 4(9):e667–e675. https://doi.org/10.1016/S2589-7500(22)00125-X.

Woo, E. J., J. Gee, P. Marquez, J. Baggs, W. E. Abara, M. M. McNeil, R. B. Dimova, and J. R. Su. 2023. Post-authorization safety surveillance of AD.26.CoV2.S vaccine: Reports to the Vaccine Adverse Event Reporting System and V-safe, February 2021–February 2022. *Vaccine* 41(30):4422–4430. https://doi.org/10.1016/j.vaccine.2023.06.023.

Xu, S., R. Huang, L. S. Sy, S. Glenn, D. S. Ryan, K. Morrissette, D. Shay, G. Vazquez-Benitez, J. M. Glanz, N. P. Klein, D. L. McClure, E. Liles, E. Weintraub, H. F. Tseng, and L. Qian. 2021. COVID-19 vaccination and non–COVID-19 mortality risk—seven integrated health care organizations, United States, December 14, 2020–July 31, 2021. *MMWR* 70. https://doi.org/10.15585/mmwr.mm7043e2.

Xu, S., R. Huang, L. S. Sy, V. Hong, S. C. Glenn, D. S. Ryan, K. Morrissette, G. Vazquez-Benitez, J. M. Glanz, and N. P. Klein. 2023. A safety study evaluating non-COVID-19 mortality risk following COVID-19 vaccination. *Vaccine* 41(3):844–854. https://doi.org/10.1016/j.vaccine.2022.12.036.

Xu, S., L. S. Sy, V. Hong, P. Farrington, S. C. Glenn, D. S. Ryan, A. M. Shirley, B. J. Lewin, H.-F. Tseng, and G. Vazquez-Benitez. 2024. Mortality risk after COVID-19 vaccination: A self-controlled case series study. *Vaccine* 42(7):1731–1737. https://doi.org/10.1016/j.vaccine.2024.02.032.

Yih, W. K., M. F. Daley, J. Duffy, B. Fireman, D. McClure, J. Nelson, L. Qian, N. Smith, G. Vazquez-Benitez, and E. Weintraub. 2023a. A broad assessment of COVID-19 vaccine safety using tree-based data-mining in the Vaccine Safety Datalink. *Vaccine* 41(3):826–835. https://doi.org/10.1016/j.vaccine.2022.12.026.

Yih, W. K., M. F. Daley, J. Duffy, B. Fireman, D. McClure, J. Nelson, L. Qian, N. Smith, G. Vazquez-Benitez, and E. Weintraub. 2023b. Tree-based data mining for safety assessment of first COVID-19 booster doses in the Vaccine Safety Datalink. *Vaccine* 41(2):460–466. https://doi.org/10.1016/j.vaccine.2022.11.053.

Yih, W. K., M. F. Daley, J. Duffy, B. Fireman, D. L. McClure, J. C. Nelson, L. Qian, N. Smith, G. Vazquez-Benitez, E. Weintraub, J. T. B. Williams, S. Xu, and J. C. Maro. 2023c. Safety signal identification for COVID-19 bivalent booster vaccination using tree-based scan statistics in the Vaccine Safety Datalink. *Vaccine* 41(36):5265–5270. https://doi.org/10.1016/j.vaccine.2023.07.010.

Yih, W. K., J. Duffy, J. R. Su, S. Bazel, B. Fireman, L. Hurley, J. C. Maro, P. Marquez, P. Moro, and N. Nair. 2024. Tinnitus after COVID-19 vaccination: Findings from the Vaccine Adverse Event Reporting System and the Vaccine Safety Datalink. *American Journal of Otolaryngology* 45(6):104448. https://doi.org/10.1016/j.amjoto.2024.104448.

Yousaf, A. R., M. M. Cortese, A. W. Taylor, K. R. Broder, M. E. Oster, J. M. Wong, A. Y. Guh, D. W. McCormick, S. Kamidani, and E. P. Schlaudecker. 2022. Reported cases of multisystem inflammatory syndrome in children aged 12–20 years in the USA who received a COVID-19 vaccine, December, 2020, through August, 2021: A surveillance investigation. *Lancet Child & Adolescent Health* 6(5):303–312. https://doi.org/10.1016/S2352-4642(22)00028-1.

Zhou, Z.-H., M. M. Cortese, J.-L. Fang, R. Wood, D. S. Hummell, K. A. Risma, A. E. Norton, M. KuKuruga, S. Kirshner, and R. L. Rabin. 2023. Evaluation of association of anti-PEG antibodies with anaphylaxis after mRNA COVID-19 vaccination. *Vaccine* 41(28):4183–4189. https://doi.org/10.1016/j.vaccine.2023.05.029.